The Carpathia Health Plan

The Rescue Healthcare Delivery System for America

Robert Dennis, MD

Published by Robert Dennis, M.D., P.A.

Photo credits: RMS Carpathia: Everett Historical/Shutterstock.com; Titanic survivors aboard lifeboat, courtesy of The National Archives and Records Administration.

www.carpathiahealthplan.com

Cataloging-in-Publication data on file with the Library of Congress

ISBN: 978-0-9974240-5-8
The Carpathia Health Plan

Printed in the United States of America.

Preface

Why Carpathia?

The Carpathia was the only ship that came to the Titanic's rescue and saved 705 doomed passengers.

The story of the RMS Carpathia is one of the most compelling rescues in maritime history. Shortly after midnight on April 15, 1912, the Carpathia's wireless operator, Harold Cottam, received an urgent message from the RMS Titanic. The renowned "unsinkable" ship had struck an iceberg and was in need of immediate assistance. Cottam woke ship Captain Arthur Henry Rostron to alert him to the distress call. Captain Rostron took swift action to ensure that the Carpathia would reach the doomed Titanic as quickly as possible. He ordered all steam to be diverted from the ship's heating system to the engines to increase the ship's speed. He also had his crew prepare for the rescued passengers, even before he knew there would be any.

As the Carpathia raced through the frigid, icy North Atlantic, the Titanic disaster continued to unfold. Although some fortunate passengers did board the limited number of available lifeboats, once the Titanic began to rapidly sink, hundreds of passengers and crew fell or jumped from the ship and landed in the freezing water. Many of them died on or just after impact.

The Carpathia reached Titanic's 20 lifeboats at 4am, and the crew quickly began pulling the survivors to the safety of their ship. Captain Rostron's immediate and deliberate decisions saved 705 Titanic passengers. But more than 1500 others had perished.

Our healthcare delivery system is sinking.

The blueprint created here to rescue our current healthcare delivery system is much like the RMS Carpathia. Our current healthcare delivery system is in nearly the same state as the Titanic during the early morning hours of April 15, 1912, nearly ready to break apart and sink to the depths. Like the Carpathia, this proposal aims **to take immediate action** to swiftly reach the health care consumers who are currently stranded by the faltering existing system.

Robert Dennis, MD

This proposal is intended to be politically neutral.

About the Author

Robert Dennis, MD is an orthopaedic surgeon who has practiced medicine for 40 years. He established and developed an orthopaedic surgery practice in Monmouth County, New Jersey, and maintained long-term affiliations with several hospitals in the New York metropolitan area, serving as Director of Orthopaedic Surgery at Jersey Shore University Medical Center, Neptune, NJ.

Dr. Dennis is passionate about his work as a physician, surgeon, inventor, teacher, lecturer and researcher. During the progression of his career, he has witnessed many changes in the field of medicine. But in recent years, the intrusion of government has dramatically increased.

The wide sweeping developments in the U.S. healthcare system are what compelled Dr. Dennis to author, in its entirety, The Carpathia Health Plan. This proposal refutes the assumption that the American consumer is incapable of actively participating in their own medical decisions. Dr. Dennis is convinced that the exact opposite is true. This work is a testament to that truth. If adopted, this proposal will harness the individual's proven capabilities to assess value and quality in the deployment of their healthcare dollar just as they do in every other interaction.

Table of Contents

Introduction

This book explains in detail a new and innovative concept in healthcare delivery. Its implementation can be partial or gradual, but the rescue is urgent.

The Carpathia Health Plan accomplishes this rescue by dismantling the bureaucratic machinery and shifting these dollars back into the delivery of actual medical care in a simple **two-step** plan:

1. Identify the six stakeholders supporting the current system.

2. Outline a slight modification in each of their roles.

The U.S. already has the most advanced and innovative medicine in the world. We need only to correct the inefficient and wasteful delivery system. We must make this correction before the entire systems sinks because of ever-escalating costs.

This effort is dedicated to those who embrace change as the path forward.

Robert Dennis, MD

January 2018

Chapter 1: Overview and Outline

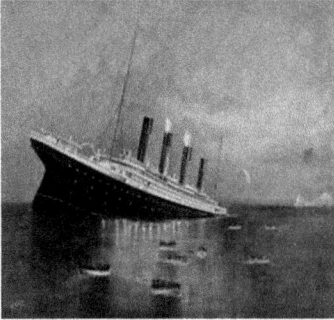

In order to obtain a health care delivery system that achieves the most desirable goals—defined as *lower costs across the system* and *full access for all*—we must be willing to consider a fundamental restructuring of the American healthcare system.

The United States healthcare system is destined for a dramatic change. The current rate of cost increases means that healthcare will cease to be available for all but a few. This is reflective of the limited lifeboats on the Titanic.

It is the universal solution and the global approach to a system in crisis. Like the RMS Carpathia, it may not stop the Titanic from sinking, but it will rescue those who are about to perish.

Outline of key elements

In order of implementation

1. Clearly define the terms **Elective Care and Urgent Care**, using already existing IDC9 codes.

2. Provide free medical care for all care defined as urgent for all people living in this country, rich or poor; funded and managed by an independent agency with government oversight.

3. Require all providers of any and all medical services to publish their fees.

4. Remove the wasteful, bureaucratic machinery that currently manages care and replace it with second opinions.

5. Require the six current stakeholders involved in healthcare delivery to make minor adjustments to their responsibilities.

   The stakeholders and their responsibilities include the following:

   A. Government:
      1. Define care as urgent or elective
      2. Establish a web-based free market platform
      3. Manage means tested insurance for low income
      4. Establish and oversee hospital outreach clinics

   B. Insurance companies:

1. Provide medical insurance based on only two parameters:
   a. Percent co-pay
   b. Second opinion threshold

C. Hospitals:
   1. Establish and manage outreach clinics
   2. Post and publish all fees for inpatient and outpatient care

D. Providers:
   1. Post and publish actual, non-inflated, direct pay fees for services and expect free market to adjust

E. Patients/Consumers
   1. Utilize shopping skills to purchase specific elective medical services
   2. Utilize second opinions in place of third-party interference; substitute second opinions for current micromanagement by third parties for every medical decision

F. Attorneys:
   1. Participate in review panel organizations following unsuccessful malpractice litigation to reduce the heavy burden that frivolous suits place on the system

Each step will be further explained in the following chapters.

Chapter 2: Basic Principles

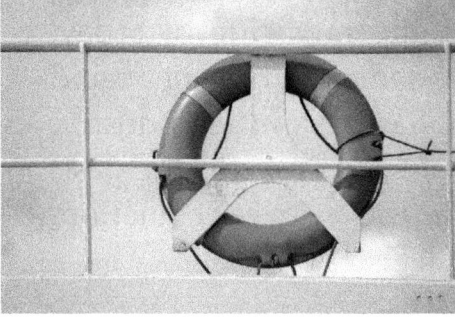

What does a test actually cost?

This is the big unknown. Most current pricing evolved from years of layered stealth negotiations between insurers and providers. This has led to artificially inflated prices for patient care visits, testing and procedures.

The Carpathia Rescue Plan will re-establish realistic and reasonable baseline pricing by allowing **providers to price care** based on their actual costs, and permit market competition to continually adjust prices.

The consumers of goods and services will have access to information that gives them the ability to evaluate cost/benefit ratios. They will be spending at least some of their own money on each unit of their own elective medical care. The free market will lower costs and improve quality of whatever product or service is being sought.

The Carpathia Health Plan remedy of substituting free and open markets for mysterious algorithms has been proven to work in cosmetic surgery, dental care, pet care, and eyewear markets. Competition has brought down prices each time. In fact, wherever it has been tried it has always demonstrated the truth of the axiom: **Appropriate competition decreases costs and increases quality.**

The Carpathia Health Plan captures the cost-lowering benefits of choice through:

- Transparency
- The improvement of quality through competition
- Access to health care for all members of society

The medicine of our fathers is not the medicine of today. Medicine has moved along the same curve of rapid advancement over the past 40 years as has every other industry. Only the structure of the delivery system is stuck in the past; buried in politics, special interests, over-regulation, bureaucracy, lobbyists, and outdated legislation.

Medicine has changed in these past 40 years and now allows the bulk of medical care to resemble other distinct flourishing consumer markets because:

1. **The consumer is smarter** and now companies directly market to consumers for complex medical products and medications on TV.
2. **Diagnoses have been well-defined** and categorized.
3. **Specific treatments have been specified for given diagnoses.**
4. The Internet's availability has permitted the consumer to become well-practiced in making web-based decisions.
5. New tools have made diagnoses more accurate and more routine, (MRI, mammogram, colonoscopy, etc.).
6. Healthcare in general is now part of all of our everyday lives:

The Carpathia Health Plan rescues the system from the two major factors that are causing it to sink.

1. The consumer has no reason to shop value versus price.

   He is not spending his own money but rather someone else's; the issue therefore changes from a cost vs. value equation to the feeling that we are all entitled to the best quality of all aspects of medicine at all times with no concern for the cost and no reason to care or shop. This is a simple and predictable result of human nature. (Certainly, this is no big surprise given the way the system is designed.)

2. The system intentionally hides the real prices of the individual goods and services in order to purposely prevent shopping and allows for the designed distortion of prices and access.

To achieve this obscuring of prices, our current healthcare system has developed thousands of new words. These terms distort, confuse and obscure the cost of what we are actually purchasing. To name just a few:

Deductibles	In-network
Copays	Out-of-network
Provider networks	Denials
Required referrals	Delays
EOBs	Maximal medical benefit
Employer-sponsored programs	IMEs
	EMRs
ERISA	Inappropriate procedure

Excessive Care
Penalties
Employer mandates
New 3.8% Medicare tax
Subsidies
Medical necessity
Waivers

Cadillac tax
Donut hole
FSA
ACO
USPSF
Advantage programs
Faith-based programs

The list goes on and on.

The more confused the consumer remains and the more docile and passive the consumer can be kept, then the longer the system can perpetuate the interests of the few power stakeholders and their profits.

Chapter 3: Rearranging the Deck Chairs

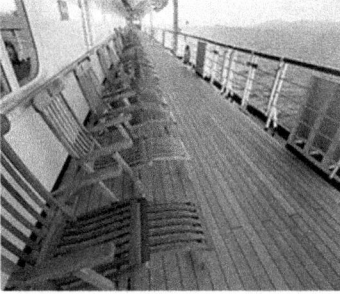

The vested interests who initially arranged the deck chairs are now scurrying to rearrange them while we all scramble for the lifeboats.

Who are the stakeholders?

There are only six total stakeholders in all.

Three are considered power players. Power players are those who most benefit from perpetuating falsely high costs:

1. **The Insurance Carriers**
2. **The Government**
3. **The Hospital Systems**

Meanwhile, the more important but far less powerful players are of course:

4. **The Patient/Consumer**
5. **The Provider (not just doctors)**
6. **The Attorneys (behind the scenes but nonetheless cost drivers)**

What's wrong with this picture?

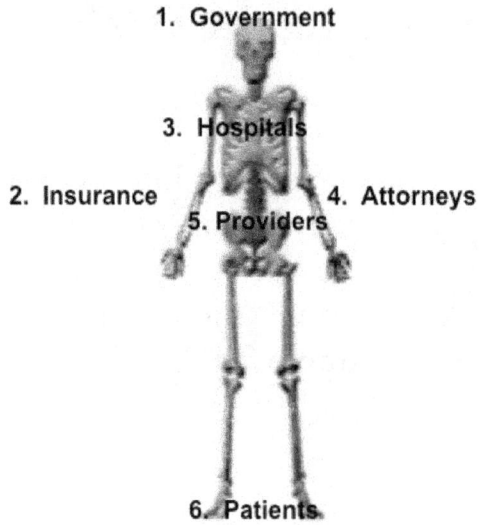

1. Government

3. Hospitals

2. Insurance   4. Attorneys

5. Providers

6. Patients

The patient should be at the top, not the
government!

Chapter 4: "Clear the Fog"

"All the things we achieve are things we have first of all imagined."

David Malouf

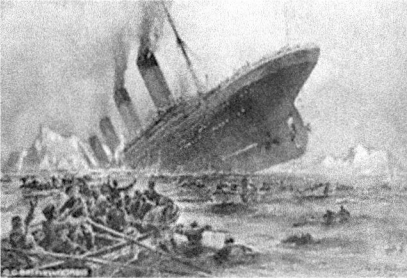

There are always new opportunities to correct mistakes and to do better. This plan promises a rescue like no other.

The Titanic sank because it hit the treacherous invisible underwater portion of the iceberg. In our current system, these hidden obstacles to medical care are the conditions threatening the system:

- Referrals
- Provider networks
- Authorizations
- Re-pricing
- Denials
- Post service denials
- Delays in payment
- Hidden taxes
- Rationing

This plan is a rescue because it guarantees:

1. Lower costs
2. Access for all people
3. Fair reimbursement
4. Less bureaucracy
5. Less unnecessary litigation
6. Any licensed provider
7. Decrease unnecessary care and waste
8. Minimize complications
9. One visible fee for every procedure

This proposal explains exactly how we can achieve these goals. It will challenge even the most adventurous among us to rethink the entire system. Had Captain Edward Smith looked below the water's surface, he might have seen the impending disaster The Titanic experienced.

Chapter 5: Before the Rescue

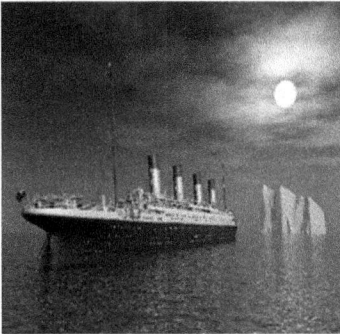

Let's examine the current typical consumer interaction in today's system. For this example, your doctor suggests you need a routine colonoscopy.

In today's system you look in your plan booklet or online provider directory and go to the provider your health insurance plan permits (the provider who accepts your insurance).

You have no other choices. You go where you are told, knowing little of the quality and nothing of the costs or the charges that a particular provider may bill your insurance company. If your co-pay is a percentage of the provider's fee, you would have no idea what that means in actual dollars since his fee is invisible to you. You do not know what the facility charge will be or what the anesthesiologist might charge. More importantly, you hope that the anesthesiologist is in your network.

In other words, as a consumer this becomes a totally blind item, as you are only responsible for the co-pay plus some unknown additional amount. At this point you have no idea of what that co-pay amount might be. You're not sure of anything, but then again they don't expect you to care about the cost, after all ... it's not your money! Or is it?

Although you now know all about the procedure because you looked it up on the Internet, you remain totally in the dark as to whether or not you really need a colonoscopy at this moment in time and how much it is really going to cost you, or your insurance company.

Now the rescue:

The Carpathia Health Plan is transparent for all elective procedures. In this example, for a colonoscopy, the website from which you would shop for the procedure, the provider and the fee might look like this:

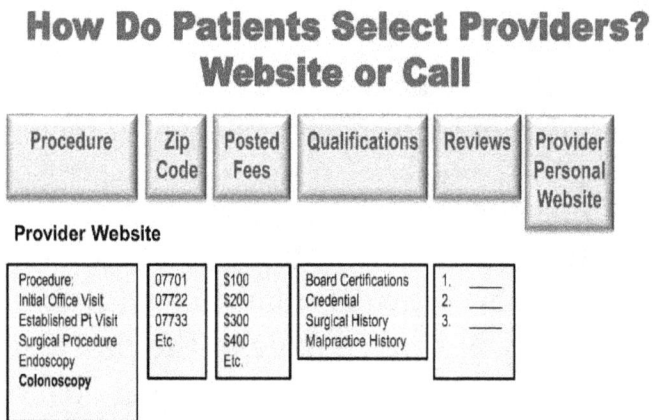

How Do Patients Select Providers?
Website or Call

Procedure	Zip Code	Posted Fees	Qualifications	Reviews	Provider Personal Website

Provider Website

Procedure: Initial Office Visit Established Pt Visit Surgical Procedure Endoscopy **Colonoscopy**	07701 07722 07733 Etc.	$100 $200 $300 $400 Etc.	Board Certifications Credential Surgical History Malpractice History	1. ___ 2. ___ 3. ___

Free market will define fees and Winners & Losers
Providers can change fees annually

Under The Carpathia Plan, when your doctor suggests that you should get a colonoscopy, the process is easy, quick, and competitive. It will entail fewer "clicks" than needed to purchase an airline ticket.

The posted fees have nothing to do with your particular insurance plan (there are no networks). These fees would be the same if you paid by cash, credit card, or any insurance plan. These fees for elective care would be the same if you had no insurance or were underinsured. These single fees would be the same if you had a green card, a blue card, or no card.

These same fees are visible to not only all consumers but also to the provider's competitors who, over a short period of time, would quickly adjust their fees to accommodate competition.

If a colleague was attracting patients, and the patient schedule of Provider "A" was full, while Provider "B" with the same credentials and qualifications was not doing so well, it would not be long before Provider "B" reduced his fee to compete effectively.

As we will explain later, in this new plan the consumer searches the procedure website for the desired procedure, identifies his ZIP Code, and searches for a provider of his choice based on quality and price. (Both the provider search and the procedure search website would be similar.) This would only take a few clicks. All willing licensed providers would be listed. Each website field would be individually searchable via drop down menus.

There are no networks, no referrals needed, no artificial state line restrictions, no third party in the room between you and your provider and nothing prohibiting you from shopping several providers or prohibiting consumers from shopping several insurance companies.

Three clicks later, you select the provider of your choice at the price you wish to pay and make an appointment.

Some may want the cheapest, some consumers may want the most expensive, some consumers may want the best by credentials and feedback, and some consumers may not care or just want the closest.

It's your choice!

In the Carpathia Health Plan (CHP), the annual repurchase of health insurance is even easier than finding a provider, and even more transparent. The consumer first assesses his likelihood of anticipated medical utilization expected in the coming year. In this new plan, the consumer then selects the co-pay percentage with which he is comfortable.

The website which he would then purchase health insurance would look something like this:

User Friendly Window for Consumer Insurance.
How Do Patients Select Insurance?

Percent Co-pay (PC)	Second Opinion Threshold (SOT)	ZIP Code	Compare Price
Consumer Selects	Consumer Selects		
10% PC 15% PC 20% PC	$1,000 (SOT)	07757	$300/month Insurance Co. 1 $200/month IC 2 $150/month IC 3 x x x x IC 4 Not Available in that price range

In the Carpathia Health Plan, there are only two variables that determines the premium – percent co-pay and Second Opinion Threshold (SOT). The term SOT will be fully explained in an upcoming chapter.

All insurance companies compete exclusively on only these two variables. This strips away the confusion of limited networks, deductibles, referrals, and third-party interference between you and your doctor. Most important, it does not consider "pre-existing conditions."

The premium will vary depending on the insurance company but the consumer's choices will be simple and understandable. Please note that these issues pertain to "Elective Care" only. All urgent care is free under CHP. Life-threatening, pre-existing conditions fall outside of these selections.

However, pre-existing conditions that are non-life-threatening fall within the selection process. The consumer projects his anticipated future utilization of medical services for elective care for his known pre-existing elective conditions when he selects his percent co-pay at the time he chooses his insurance policy. The consumer, in a very transparent system, selects the insurance premium he can afford. The higher the percent co-pay he selects, the lower his premium will be (as it should be). The higher the SOT he selects, the higher his premium will be. What is new in this rescue plan is that the provider fees for all elective care are visible to the purchaser. Each individual will choose the policy that best fits his needs.

But the best part is yet to come. Let's dissect this single issue of elective care just a little further and understand the impact it will have on the cost of care for the whole system.

Because this new transparent healthcare delivery system was available, and within three clicks, your shopping effort and skill has not only saved you a considerable amount of money but it has also dramatically affected the cost of that colonoscopy to your insurer, who has to pay the other 80% or 90% of the fees.

You certainly worked no harder than you would have to get the best price and quality of a TV, refrigerator, or an airline ticket, so why not use the same intuitive and intelligent purchasing skills to purchase an elective medical procedure? The difference is that you now have access to price and quality information, much like the TV or refrigerator purchases we all make.

Let's take the example a little further so we can better understand the massive impact this simple system could have on lowering medical costs across the board.

The key is that your co-pay is a percentage of the provider's posted fee, which is now known and visible. At the annual renewal of your health care insurance policy, your healthcare insurance provider (also part of this new transparent system) offered you co-pays, as did their competitors, that ranged from 3% to 30% of the providers' posted fee. The decision was yours, according to your unique circumstances.

We assumed for the purpose of this example that you chose a 10% co-pay. The website listed several providers of colonoscopy.

1. Dr. A's posted fee was $2000, the facility where he works posted a fee of $6000, and the anesthesiologist that he works with posted a fee of $1000. To choose Dr. A meant that you would have a colonoscopy for a total cost of $9,000.

    The cost to you would be $900; this would give you the procedure performed by the doctor of your choice.

2. Dr. B's posted fee was $5000, the facility where he works posted a $10,000 fee, and the anesthesiologist (you could have chosen separately) charged $3000, for a total cost of $18,000 (double).

Robert Dennis, MD

The cost to you if you had chosen Dr. B would therefore be $1800.

You saved $900 (real money in your pocket) in this transparent system by using your shopping skills for this elective procedure.

But the best part is that you were able to provide a dramatic systemwide total cost reduction via your shopping abilities. The insurance company that sold you the policy is obligated to pay the other 90% of the provider's posted fee. You just saved your insurance company $9000. This multiplied a thousand times across the board for elective procedures gives you a glimpse of the real power and benefit of transparent competition and consumer choice. Even better is the fact that the insurance carrier had little if any bureaucratic overhead costs in this process nor did the provider. The system saved a huge amount of bureaucratic overlay. Best of all, you suffered no delays or denials.

You provided the system a huge savings and the system provided you the ability to save significantly in your medical care, while allowing you to choose your provider. It's that simple!

Multiply this one million times. Even if it doesn't work for everyone, it will certainly work for cost-conscious consumers.

The power of your shopping capabilities saved the entire system both bureaucratic and overhead costs as well as actual costs. The providers received the fee that they were willing to accept with minimal hassle. The provider and insurance carrier were freed of tremendous bureaucratic overhead and benefited from dramatically lower cost. In fact, all parties involved experience a benefit. (Currently the bureaucratic costs to deliver medical care range from 25 to 45% of the medical dollar, so these savings are no small part of getting you much more value and a much larger percentage of medical care for your medical dollar.)

Eventually all parties will benefit from the competitive marketplace by the effect that all players have on adjusting fees to realistic figures. **This portion of the envisioned healthcare program is exclusively reserved for elective care only.** Please keep in mind that the vast majority of medical costs are spent on the elective side of the ledger. Urgent or catastrophic care is free for everyone.

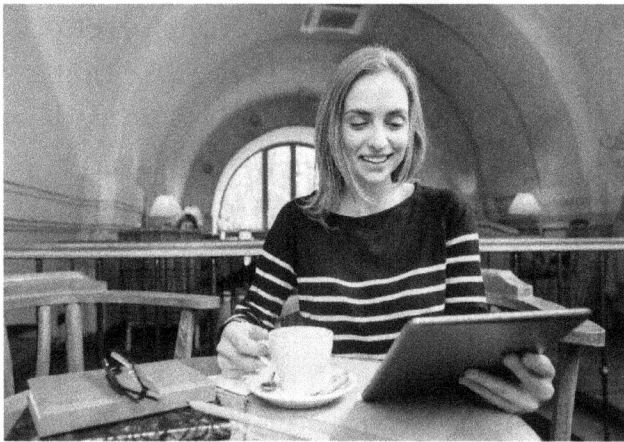

If you can shop hotels and airfare, shopping for elective care will be a piece of cake.

Chapter 6: Second Opinion for Elective Care

A Rescue From Bureaucracy

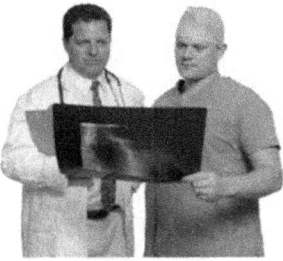

Now let's look at the other side of this equation. As an informed consumer, wouldn't you also want to ask your provider who suggested the colonoscopy why you needed it at that particular time?

A second opinion will give you more comfort than a bureaucrat in some insurance building looking at an algorithm, plugging in your age, and then sending you a denial letter.

In the Carpathia Health Plan, a second opinion rescues you from unnecessary elective procedures. In this plan it is always your option. In the CHP, second opinions are encouraged, and in some cases, even required. For example, if you had purchased insurance with a second opinion threshold of $10,000, and you were considering a very expensive procedure such as total hip replacement, a confirmatory second opinion can be required for this elective procedure.

A second opinion, by a doctor of your own choosing with qualifications at your comfort level, is a critical part of this system. The fee you might pay for the second opinion would be trivial in the scope of things (you only pay the percent co-pay of the doctor's posted fee).

A second opinion is always a good thing, and in this new system, functions as a welcome substitute for all the redundant algorithms and layered bureaucratic medicine that we all deal with currently. Please remember that your annual insurance premium has dropped from $12,000 with a deductible of $5,000 to a mere $3,000 annually because of this rescue plan.

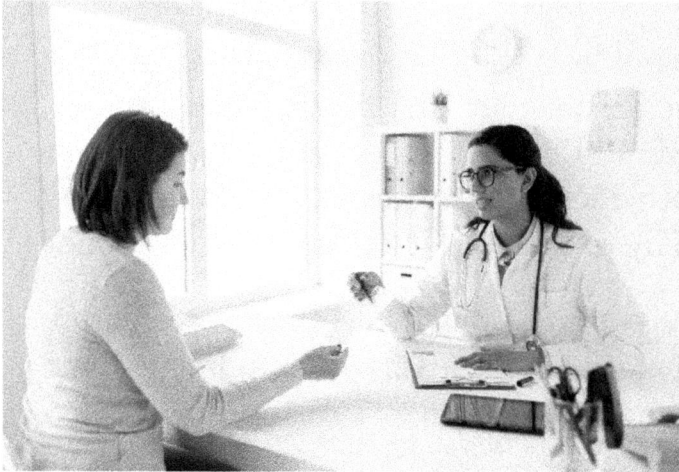

For a second opinion you would select the doctor from the same website. The website would display all the physician's qualifications and consultation fees. You would simply select the physician whose consultation fee was within your budget. Yes, of course, you have to pay the same 10% when you go for that second opinion. A second confirmatory consultation may cost perhaps $200. Your 10% co-pay would expose you to $20. A low price to pay for comfort.

You benefit with a meaningful valid second opinion which replaces piles of paperwork and unnecessary bureaucracy. This second opinion can only accrue to your benefit. If you like the second doctor, there is no prohibition, within this system, that would prevent you from staying with the second doctor, based on your comfort level.

If the second doctor agrees with the first doctor, and you decide to proceed with the procedure, the system may reward you by refunding all or a portion of the percent co-pay you expended when you proceeded with the final procedure.

On the other hand, if the second opinion doctor disagreed and opined that you did not need that procedure, but you chose to go ahead with it anyway, that is also okay; it will always be your choice. The second opinion physician is not there to prevent you from getting an appropriate procedure, but to offer an alternative opinion as a method to help you possibly avoid an unnecessary procedure.

This method of utilization review is better than any alternative algorithm or committee.

The doctor who said you need a colonoscopy or total hip procedure will know (because he also participates in the system) that you are going for a second opinion, because you have to, and therefore he may try harder to accommodate you, improve his bedside manner or shorten his wait times, even though his posted fee will continue to compete with those of his colleagues.

It will be your choice totally. This cannot hurt and is far better than the current bureaucratic method of questioning the medical necessity of every recommended elective procedure. That second consultation may save you money, time and perhaps even save you an unnecessary procedure. The second doctor may offer you an alternative option or a less dramatic pathway to wellness. This can only be a good thing for you. Most would think that the $20 would be money well spent.

Definitions & Abbreviations
What is meant by SOT?

Second Opinion Threshold = SOT:

The cost of care (as posted) over which a patient agrees to simply consult with another prescribing provider (of his choice and of the same specialty) to discuss his options in regards to a considered elective procedure, test, device, or drug.

Yes, the patient will have to pay his percent co-pay to the 2nd opinion provider (after having considered that provider's posted fee). **He gets a real 2nd opinion and the original procedures, if he so wishes**, for the price of the % co-pay.

What is missing from this entire system is deductibles, referrals, authorizations, delays and millions if not billions of dollars of administrative costs and frustration.

Chapter 7: Catastrophic Care & Conditions

No Co-pays, No SOT

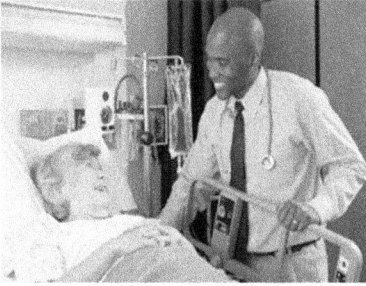

What is the best alternative for covering catastrophic care?

A balanced mix of free market transparent choice for elective procedures and a slightly more traditional approach with government oversight and participation in the cost of care for life-threatening situations. To be sure, these two separate parts of medical care need to be kept separate, thought of as separate and unique, and be clearly differentiated!

The clear definitions of urgent versus elective care is therefore the basis for the CHP. What do we mean? You can't force people into health and penalize them or their physicians if they do not make healthy life choices. You can make catastrophic care available for everyone and provide an equal playing field for all citizens/consumers as it relates to agreed upon life-threatening illness, whether self-inflicted or not.

This proposed Carpathia Health Plan will easily demonstrate enormous cost savings as it relates to catastrophic illness. It will build on the technology, diagnosis codes and procedure codes that are already well-established. It will make full use of the fraud detection systems that are already solidly in place when dealing with urgent care that limits the time needed to compare. It will be easy to roll out and will not require thousands upon thousands of confusing pages to understand.

For the purpose of overview, here are the key characteristics and benefits of the Carpathia Health Plan, in relation to serious conditions defined by the patient's diagnosis.

Carpathia Health Plan: Key Characteristics (For serious illness and urgent care):

- ✓ Covers EVERYONE – rich and poor
- ✓ Free-market driven
- ✓ Dramatically lowers healthcare costs
- ✓ New concept revolves around DEFINITIONS of elective care versus urgent and catastrophic care (rather than mandates and penalties)
- ✓ Easy to understand and implement
- ✓ Enhances patient choice and the doctor/patient relationship
- ✓ Assumes that both rich and poor are equally able to make informed healthcare decisions (in the same way we decide which TV, food, or appliance to purchase) – value versus price (we are good at this)
- ✓ Relies on legitimate second opinions instead of rationing committees, government penalties, subsidies, referrals, authorizations, provider networks, deductibles and bureaucratic obstructions

Chapter 8: The System's Linchpin

The Critical Line Between Urgent Care and Elective Care

The critical line that makes this system work is a line that is already well-established and easily understood in medicine and can be quickly formalized and detailed.

It is the line between acute care and elective care.

The definition of acute care is simply any care that addresses any life-threatening or limb-threatening issue.

Examples of life or limb-threatening care:

- Catastrophic care
- Cancer care
- Acute cardiac care including cardiac catheterization, stents and angioplasties
- Acute pulmonary care
- Fracture care

Anything that threatens life or limb either in the short-term or long-term, including a situation/condition in which delayed treatment might jeopardize life or limb.

The exact, well laid-out and fully described definition of such care will be left to specialty experts and government panels, and will be modifiable from time to time and published for all to see by a government panel set up within the Carpathia Health Plan. There will be a built-in place for meaningful feedback and recommendations that will allow for improvement over time.

The definition of elective care is very simple: all other care that is not defined above. (Most money is spent on the elective care portion of medical costs.)

Examples of elective care:

- Any care that can wait or is non-urgent
- Any routine testing or exams
- Long-term management of illnesses such as diabetes or arthritis
- Anything that can wait without incurring dire consequences (anything where there is sufficient time for a second opinion; a condition that might have gone on for any length of time and where allowing it to go on for some additional time will not be detrimental to the patient)
- Such procedures as MRIs, CT scans
- Arthroscopies
- Total hip replacements
- Total knee replacements
- Pain management
- Most psychiatric issues, etc.

When a diagnosis changes from one defined within the group of "elective care" to one that falls under the "urgent care" definition, the coverage and payment method changes to full coverage paid through a different funding source with no contributions required from the patient. In other words, the treatment becomes completely free and fully available to all inhabitants of this country.

The payor changes when the diagnosis changes.

Examples:

- Headache to brain tumor
- Cold to pneumonia
- Weakness to stroke
- Pre-diabetes to diabetes
- Depression to schizophrenia

The patient responsibilities also change when the diagnosis changes.

How is the <u>Definition of Elective Care &</u> Urgent/Catastrophic Decided?

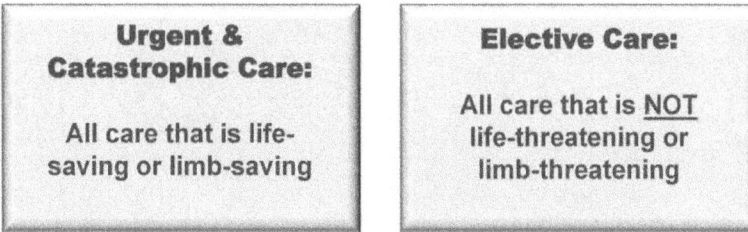

Urgent & Catastrophic Care: All care that is life-saving or limb-saving	Elective Care: All care that is <u>NOT</u> life-threatening or limb-threatening

✓ Each specialty lists which diagnosis and which procedures (using current codes) are life-saving and limb-saving in their specialty

✓ HHS approves the lists and publishes the list on the web and in hard copy to all providers and public (revisable every 2 years)

Chapter 9: Abbreviations and Terms

To assist in the understanding of some specific terms that will be repeated in this overview, please take a close look at the following terms and definitions:

Summary of Abbreviations
To be used in this concept

P   = Provider

PF = Posted Fee

PC = % Co-pay

SOT = Second Opinion Threshold

EC = Elective Care

UC = Urgent & Catastrophic Care

UC = Urgent Care or catastrophic care or emergency care has already been well defined as life-threatening, limb-threatening life-limiting.

EC = Elective Care has already been well described in previous chapters.

P = Provider refers to any and all medical providers, not just physicians but also nurses, hospitals, chiropractors, EMTs, clinics and surgery centers, etc.

Definitions & Abbreviations

Posted Fees = PF

Those fees required to be posted by **every** provider for **all** the goods and services they provide on **all** published schedules in the order of frequency provided. Providers set their own fees and will **compete** in the marketplace for price with other providers of the same service in their same **zip code**. (They can change their fees annually based on supply and demand.)

% Copay = PC:

The percent of the posted fee that the patient has selected (when he chooses his insurance) that he agrees to pay to the provider.

OR

The percent copay that was assigned to him/her by a uniform means test at the hospital outreach clinic.

Definitions & Abbreviations
What is meant by SOT?

Second Opinion Threshold = SOT:

The cost of care (as posted) over which a patient agrees to simply consult with another prescribing provider (of his choice and of the same specialty) to discuss his options in regards to a considered elective procedure, test, device, or drug.

Yes, the patient will have to pay his percent co-pay to the 2nd opinion provider (after having considered that provider's posted fee). **He gets a real 2nd opinion and the original procedures, if he so wishes**, for the price of the % co-pay.

What is missing from this entire system is deductibles, referrals, authorizations, delays and millions if not billions of dollars of administrative costs and frustration.

Understanding these simple new terms represents all that will be required in order to understand the entire concept.

Please refer to these pages as we go into more detail, utilizing these abbreviations to easily and visually explain the actuarial assumptions that provide for the funding as well as a full explanation and implementation of this plan.

Chapter 10: The Role of Government

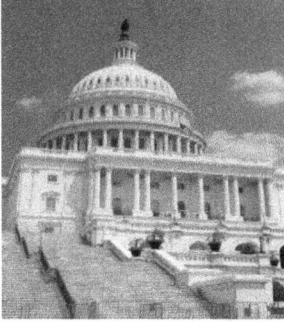

The role of government will be several-fold, as follows:

1. **To create** and continually update the definitions of life-threatening or limb-threatening listed procedures utilizing well-established diagnoses and procedure codes.

2. **To define** and continually update a nationally published, per state, means test to be applied to uninsured and underinsured residents. A simple actuarial derived graph of income versus percent co-pay and confirmatory second opinion threshold that hospital intake centers would apply uniformly to individual patients applying for assisted or government coverage. This will be explained in more detail in later chapters.

3. **Establish and oversee the outreach clinics** required to be established by each hospital to care for the underinsured and uninsured patients that have acquired an assisted or government coverage insurance card.

4. **Establish and maintain fraud and abuse guidelines** in appropriate places within the system, many of which have already been well-identified.

5. **Establish and maintain national informational**

public websites with secure provider portals. Through one website, providers can list the fees that they will accept for all the procedures that they do in the order of frequency. A second website provides complete information on the credentials, qualifications, licenses, procedure histories, malpractice history and patient feedback ratings of each provider. These websites are to be available to all.

Given that the government is already experienced with the intricacies of setting up a website and have by now learned the process well, one might anticipate that these challenges would not be overwhelming.

How Does Assigned Insurance Work?

Go to Hospital &/or Hospital Outreach Clinic Intake/Reception

Sum of All Sources of Income	Proof of Income	Zip	Sign Fraud Statement	Means PC	Means SOT
____ $____ ____ $____ ____ $____ Total $____	_____ _____ _____ _____	_____	"I affirm under penalty of the law..." Yes ____ No ____	_____ _____ _____ _____	_____ _____ _____ _____

Who Can Apply for Assigned Insurance?
Anyone or Everyone

Means tested income will likely produce higher PC & SOT than private carriers for wealthier patients

Chapter 11: The Six Stakeholders

Government

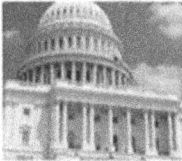

Hospitals

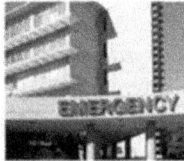

Insurance Companies

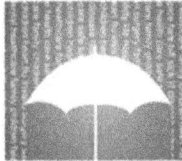

Attorneys

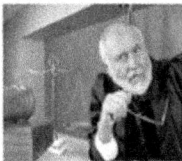

Providers

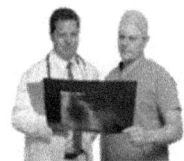

Consumers

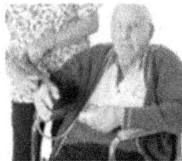

It is important to acknowledge that healthcare delivery is substantially affected by six unique participants, all of whom have reason to want to protect their own interest or turf. However, any serious effort to reform health care has to identify and to some extent modify the manner in which all six of these participants impact the system.

There is a reason that we dedicated this book to those who embrace change as the path forward. Change is the hardest request we can make of any individual.

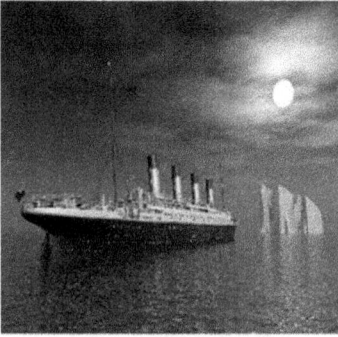

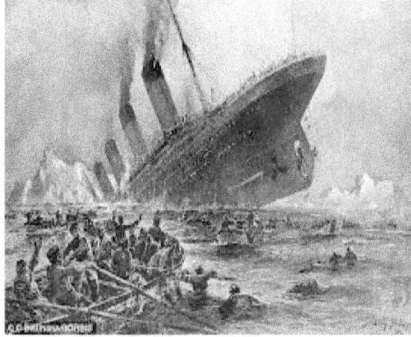

If Titanic had changed course, the disaster may have been avoided.

Any change in the system must incorporate and require change in the way all six participants provide and receive benefit. We have previously identified the six players and separated the three power players from the non-power players in the roles that they currently hold. Understand that none of the players who have already staked out positions in the current system will invite a change that will alter roles that they had so ardently fought for. But change must come because the system is sinking before our eyes, no longer providing health care in the way we need to receive it. Future generations should not be asked to pay for our unwillingness to act.

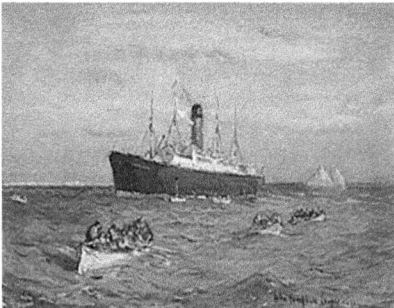

The Carpathia Health Plan represents a sea change in the manner that healthcare delivery will be carried out. Therefore, one must anticipate full-fledged resistance in the form of detailed criticism of every aspect of this reform. However, for the better good it is hoped that all six players will be able to look beyond their specific prejudices and appreciate that they are being asked to change on an equal basis. Some will acknowledge beneficial change as it applies to the other five, and some will scream that the changes that apply to them are negative. However, if all six players are willing to think out of the box, then the system will benefit everyone, and their own benefits will ultimately far surpass the changes they are being asked to consider individually.

We will describe these changes in the form of new rules for each stakeholder.

We previously detailed the role that the government would play in this new system. Next, we will examine all six players and describe the role modification required for each one. When taken together, a dramatic new system will emerge from the current shattered and dysfunctional system.

The players in order of importance are:

1. The Patient

2. The Provider

3. The Hospitals

4. The Insurance Carriers

5. The Government

6. The Attorneys

We must think of each stakeholder as a rower on a life boat. Each must do their part if the passengers are going to be saved.

ALL SIX PLAYERS WILL BE AFFECTED BY CHANGE

1. New Rules
2. Advantages
3. Disadvantages
4. Medicare to be untouched for 10 years

However, purely for the purposes of better understanding of the system, we will present the changes that each player must make so that the reader can best understand the whole picture.

New Rules and Details
Each Stakeholder will be affected

1. Government
2. Insurance Companies
3. Hospitals
4. Attorneys
5. Providers
6. Patients

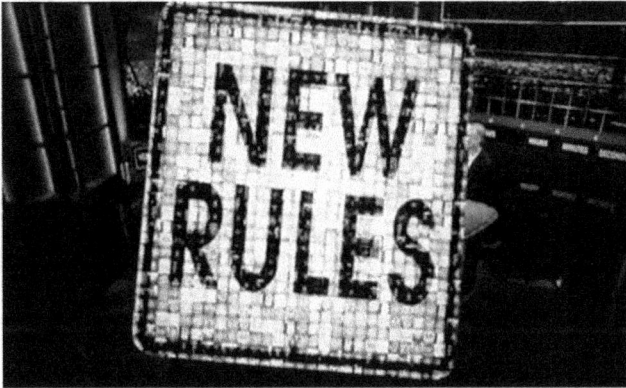

GOVERNMENT: New Rules

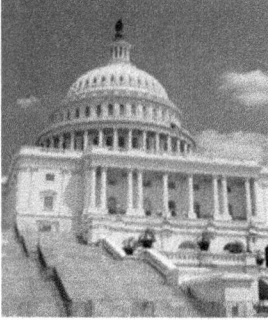

1. Clearly provide the definitions of urgent, catastrophic, and elective care

2. Fund in large measure two distinct pools of money (that any provider or hospital can access if the care provided meets the definitions): **Urgent and/or Catastrophic Pool** and **Uninsured Pool**

3. Define a Universal Means Test that is zip code specific

4. Set up and manage two large comprehensive websites: **Provider Fees and Provider Qualifications**

Details: Government

A. Fully and clearly define **terms** (for all to know and abide by)

    1. **Catastrophic**, urgent (life-saving or limb-saving care), which combined presently represent the smaller portion of medical costs.

2. **Non-urgent** care, which is **ALL** care not defined as **urgent** or **catastrophic**. (This currently represents the majority of medical costs.)

3. **All care** determined to be catastrophic care is to be paid for by the catastrophic care pool for all patients whether they have insurance or not (without having to pay any co-pay). The fund will pay 100% of such care.

4. The means test that clinics and hospitals use to delineate what amount uninsured patients who appear for care at hospital outreach clinics will have to pay, if anything.

5. Define "practical frivolous lawsuits" exclusively for medical malpractice cases (see **Attorneys**). (Litigation that failed and that has been found to be frivolous by both medical and legal peer review panels as will be described in a later chapter.)

B. **LEAVE MEDICARE ALONE:** Tax whoever you have to, but do it transparently and identify the source of revenues.

C. Investigate and prosecute cases of suspected fraud, system abuse, or over-treatment especially as related to medical/legal cases and other types of criminal behavior that constitute stealing from the system. (Laws are already in place but not vigorously enforced.)

D. Design and manage two important websites that will include **ALL** providers of medical care. **One for fees and one for qualifications**; both sorted by any of several variables.

E. Lift prohibition against suing HMOs.

F. Fund, in combination with state government, hospital-run outreach clinics through an **"Uninsured Care Pool."**

This pool will be funded by a combination of contributions from:

- Federal Government
- State Government
- Private Insurance companies
- Philanthropic Organizations
- Patients who access these hospital outreach clinics according to a uniformly applied "means test"

G. Fund, in combination with insurance carriers and state governments, a pool titled **"Catastrophic Care Pool."**

H. The government must clearly identify the revenue sources and taxes being levied to support this "Uninsured Care Pool" as well as the "Catastrophic Care Pool."

I. Expand and devise health saving plans for employees **and individuals.**

J. Extend COBRA and provide tax credit for individuals who purchase healthcare insurance to the same extent as groups of employees enjoy when they purchase health care through their employers. (This biased government tax supplement should be removed so the playing field can be equalized and blind to where the insurance was purchased.)

K. Enact tort reform as described in the section titled "Attorneys."

L. Direct and regulate hospitals and patients to abide by definitions of catastrophic and urgent care. Require hospital emergency rooms to direct all care determined to be **"non-urgent care" to their outreach clinics or to the patients' private doctors.**

This will allow hospital Emergency Rooms to take care of only urgent and catastrophic care and redirect all other care. This will save millions and yet provide appropriate care to both the uninsured and the insured.

INSURANCE COMPANIES:

New Rules

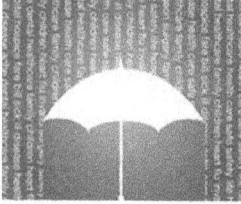

1. Pay for second opinions, both voluntary and mandatory, to replace utilization review. This will eliminate the need for referrals, authorizations, deductibles, denials, and provider networks. The huge insurance company bureaucracies will be retired.

2. Establish competitive premiums on the basis of only two parameters:

   a. The amount of percent co-pay the patient chooses

   b. The threshold level that triggers a mandatory specialty-specific second opinion (or SOT)

Details: Insurance Companies

A. Provide catastrophic insurance separately delineated as a specific portion of the premium charged and provide such catastrophic funds to the National Catastrophic Pool. Based on some proportion to be shared with the government and other voluntary supporters, **this pool will pay for all catastrophic care.**

B. Pay 100% of all care of their insureds that fits the government definition of urgent care with no co-pay or no second opinions necessary via its contribution to the **Urgent Care Fund**, seen as a line item on each insured's annual premium invoice.

Provide a portion of their premium (line item, clear and transparent) for uninsured care to go to a pool along with government funds to support hospital outreach clinics to cover their share of medical care for the poor. This pool will receive insurance company funds as well as government funds and patient payments (based on a uniform means test) as well as charitable contributions.

C. Provide insurance coverage for all elective care of their insureds, minus a 1% to 30% co-pay (depending on the specific policy). Co-pays are to be paid on all bills where elective care is provided. (No care can be completely free if a patient has insurance. We all must have "skin in the game.") Even if the co-pay is very small, it must be applied to all bills.

Insurance companies will sell policies on the basis of only two criteria:
   1. Percent of co-pay the patient chooses for elective care;
   2. Second Opinion Threshold (SOT)

Summary: Insurance companies will compete on two key parameters:

1. Premiums associated with a given co-pay, 1% to 30%. The higher the co-pay, the smaller the premium.

2. Premiums associated with a patient-selected second opinion threshold (SOT). The lower the threshold, the lower the premium.

3. All urgent care provided at 0% co-pay.

4. Insurance companies will require patients to pay only a discounted portion of their selected co-pay, whatever that is, to hospitals or surgicenters for non-urgent care (to protect patients/consumers from huge bills).

5. Insurance companies will pay 100% of urgent care costs.

HOSPITALS & SURGICENTERS: New Rules

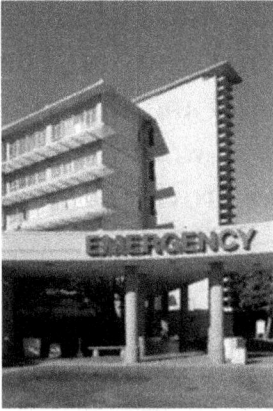

1. ER Triage will have authority to direct ER patients for treatment and admission, or direct all other patients to outreach clinics (not necessarily their own) or private care, clearly based on the diagnosis and definition criteria.

2. Post all fees (simplified and unbundled).

3. Bill appropriate fund for care that fits the appropriate definition and appropriately collect the adjusted co-pay or means-tested fee.

4. Leave Medicare alone for now.

5. Hospitals are required to set up and run outreach clinics for non-urgent care. All clinic fees are to be posted. Clinics will compete with other local hospital outreach clinics.

6. Pay all providers that work in their clinics their posted fees in full.

Item 6 above represents a benefit to providers. The provider (physician) who can charge only one fee (the fee posted) whenever he performs a specific service will earn more when he performs that same service in the hospital clinic setting. The provider will be paid that same fee by the hospital and will earn more by working in the hospital clinic than they would if they performed that service in their own office. (The provider incurs no overhead while working in the clinic.)

As a result, the hospital will have no problem recruiting medical talent to work in the clinic. Doctors will compete for these positions.

Details: Hospitals

A. All hospitals will establish and run outreach clinics funded by the government via a specific formula. (Many already have.) This will provide for incredible savings by reducing the overloads in emergency rooms while at the same time providing appropriate and timely care to all people; not much different from what occurs now, but with much less waste of resources.

B. These clinics will:

1. Cover all specialties provided in the hospitals.

2. Provide only non-urgent care.

3. Care for all people with and without insurance. Co-pays apply if the patient has insurance. A means test will apply in place of a co-pay if the patient has no insurance.

4. Provide a uniform **means test** to all patients so they pay according to what they can afford.

5. Post their clinic fees for care like all other providers.

6. Charge the same fees as they posted and pay their doctors the fees that the doctors have posted.

7. Obligate providers and their staff to man these clinics. Since providers will be paid the same fees that they receive in their private practice (the fees that they posted), serving in these clinics will actually be desirable since the doctors will have less overhead.

C. The funding formula for these clinics can be a combination of:

1. Federal government funding, perhaps 50%.

2. Private insurance funding from a pool (like uninsured motorists) listed separately as an identified portion of everyone's premium, perhaps 10% labeled "uninsured care."

3. Charitable contributions from individuals and charitable organizations (fully tax deductible to donor).

4. State government. (All revenue sources designated by federal and state governments clearly identified and transparent)

D. Hospitals will now be able to redirect non-urgent care to their outreach clinics and unload their Emergency Rooms, and still make some profit from their outreach clinics. The outreach clinics will compete with each other.

ATTORNEYS: New Rules

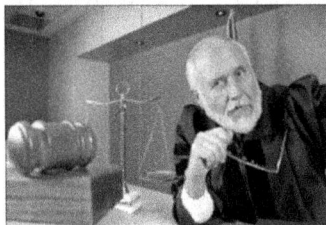

1. New national caps on pain and suffering.

2. Submit apparent frivolous LOST malpractice cases to the scrutiny of:

   a. Medical Peer Review Process

   b. Legal Peer Review Process

3. Be subjected to nominal penalties if all three processes (litigation and Peer Reviews) result in detrimental findings.

Details: Attorneys

Two pathways to real tort reform.

Fact 1: 30% of tests and care are originated by doctors who feel that they have to protect themselves from malpractice litigation.

Fact 11: 15% of providers as well as hospital fees are devoted to cover malpractice premiums.

Legislation 1: Caps on pain and suffering

Suggested awards from $250,000 to $450,000, with full reimbursement for true losses (wages, future care, etc.). This has been tried and has worked in every state where it has been tried.

Legislation 2: Penalties for filing frivolous malpractice lawsuits

1. Penalties not to exceed the true court costs (the waste of judicial time). Penalties are necessary; however, they must be fair.

2. Penalties to be split in reverse of contingency fee. (If the lawyer agrees upon a win, take 30% of the proceeds from the case. Then the lawyer is to pay 70% of the penalty and the patient pays 30% if the case is determined to be frivolous.)

3. The government is to create a new practical definition of frivolous which is different from the legal definition. Call it "Practical Frivolous" and let it be covered by the attorney's malpractice insurance:

   a. This new definition of frivolous is made up of three criteria. All three must be confirmed frivolous and all three must be in agreement with each other.

   Criteria #1: Lose the litigation. Had to be lost before a jury (no cause verdict).

   Criteria #2: Medical Peer Review Panel must find that the **provider was not at fault**. Panel to be selected randomly from a pool, outside of the jurisdiction of the medical provider that was sued, and made up of three defense medical experts and three plaintiff medical experts and one randomly selected blindly from the same pool of an equal number of defense and plaintiff experts.

Criteria #3: Legal Peer Review made up of a panel of three randomly selected defense attorneys and three plaintiff attorneys and one selected blindly from the same pool of an equal number of defense and plaintiff attorneys. Each panel of attorneys to be selected from different jurisdictions and freshly appointed for each case. (Very similar to Medical Peer Review)

4. All expert witness testimony in all malpractice cases is to be published on the Internet and reviewed for scientific validity; review comments permitted on website.

Periodic review of the comments to be undertaken by each state medical licensing board who will consider disciplinary action against expert witnesses if certain high threshold criteria are met and where truthful evidence-based and scientifically supported testimony is brought into question.

5. Lift prohibition against suing HMOs.

6. Substantial penalties should be imposed **for encouraging clients** to seek unnecessary medical treatment to enhance their probability of winning their litigation. Prosecution should be initiated against the attorney as would occur in any other criminal case for conspiracy to commit insurance fraud.

PROVIDERS: New Rules

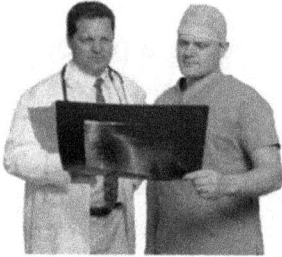

1. Post and annually update fees and qualifications on government website.

2. Agree to have one and only one fee for each service.

3. Disseminate fees upon request and post fees in the office.

4. Collect co-pays or means-tested fees from all patients.

5. Bill all urgent/catastrophic care to the appropriate pool (no co-pay). You will be paid 100% of your fee every time.

6. Be available and affirm the second opinion requirement when indicated.

Details: Providers—doctors, hospitals, physical therapists, chiropractors, etc. (all providers)

A. Require **all providers** of medical services to:
   1. Post all of their fees and charge only those fees to all patients and all payers (using descriptions and current codes).

a. Make all fees easy to understand. (Like all other commodities)

b. Agree to have one and only one fee for each service.

c. Describe all fees in pamphlets, faxes, waiting room, posters, websites, etc. (all fees must be in a meaningful order of frequency).

d. Describe all fees in the order of their most common services to their least common services.

e. Post the single most appropriate, fair, reasonable, and realistic fee that they must accept for that given service and that they expect to be paid each time they perform that service regardless of who they bill or who ends up paying. (No one will set these fees but them.) Each provider will then quickly adjust to the true market forces of supply and demand.

   The law of supply and demand will quickly take over.

f. Agree to provide their fees to all patients at all times and most importantly before their appointment and require signature of the patient (like HIPAA).

g. Utilize already established CPT codes with the same unbundling rules that currently apply.

h. Re-affirm or change their fees on an annual basis.

i. Understand all laws to end price fixings as it affects them and expect to be prosecuted if found guilty.

2. Post their qualifications: credentials, malpractice history, practice history, most frequently performed procedures, complication rate, etc.

3. Post fees and qualifications on uniform, sortable websites to be maintained by the government.

4. Be responsible to verify and update their information annually.

5. Expect to be prosecuted for conspiracy to commit insurance fraud in cases where practice patterns reflect abuse or excessive treatment, particularly when litigation or entitlement programs are liable for medical bills. (Enhanced prosecution of medical, legal mills.)

6. Bill all care defined to be catastrophic care to catastrophic pool.

This plan will eliminate pre-authorization/precertification and referrals, along with all the bureaucracy and associated costs.

PATIENTS: New Rules

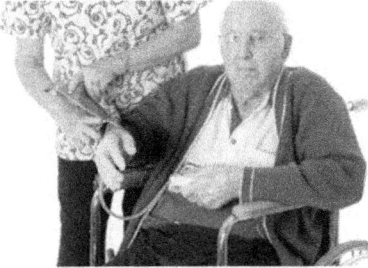

Patients will be expected to:

1. Shop insurance policies based on only two variable parameters:

    a. Amount of co-pay (% of fees)

    b. Dollar amount of threshold for second opinion (the lower the threshold, the lower the premium)

2. Pay their share of the co-pay or means test for every piece of elective care (skin in the game).

3. Shop and purchase all elective medical care based on transparent and easily available cost and quality parameters.

4. If they have no insurance, select a hospital-run outreach clinic and be means tested for all elective care (the means test could require the patient to pay as little as 0.5% or 0% of all care).

5. Obtain and abide by the required second opinions.

Details: Patients (Below age 65)

A. Will be **required** to obtain second opinions for all non-urgent procedures over a certain amount; with no restrictions on a patient switching doctors. (Good for patients, good for doctors and good for the system.)

   1. Patients to select the second opinion doctor for consultation in the same way and for the same posted fee as the patient selected the first doctor.

   2. Patients select their second opinion threshold amount when they purchase their insurance. This will vary according to their choice. (The higher the threshold, the higher the premium; the lower the threshold amount, the lower their insurance premium.) Insurance companies will want to encourage second opinions as a means of lowering their costs.

B. Shop for cost and quality to save their own money (via co-pay) in the same way as they would shop for any other item; by becoming knowledgeable and shopping price vs. quality (all of which is now readily available to them and will lower costs enormously).

Summary: The need for pre-authorizations/pre-certifications, primary care referrals, as well as all other paperwork and delays will be eliminated. This will in turn eliminate the bureaucracy and associated costs. All catastrophic care will be billed to the catastrophic fund with 0% co-pay to the patient. All urgent care will be paid for by their insurance company via their contribution to the Urgent Care Fund with 0% co-pay to the patient.

This chapter has summarized the new obligations and

responsibilities of each of the six participants. By redefining the roles of all six, the cost of the entire conglomerate of healthcare goods and services will be dramatically reduced.

We can anticipate enormous resistance to change. Each stakeholder is expected to vigorously object and find endless reasons why this dramatic new concept can't work. However, when one looks at it from an overview, it is simple and no more than the way it would have evolved had it not been for the political interference of each of the six participants. The current crisis is the result of the layered bureaucracy created over time. We believe it is time to correct these distortions.

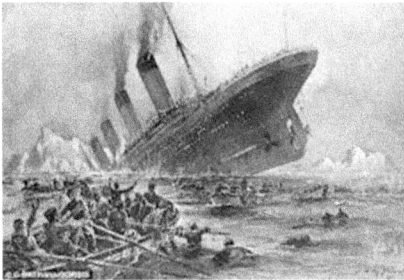

If the system is allowed to continue without rescue, we will all suffer, as will our children.

Chapter 12: Tax Reductions, Not Increases

This may be hard for industry experts to fathom. One can understand the effect that 40 years of piled on paperwork and bureaucratic administration has had on all of us.

However, all we need to do is add up the current **total** healthcare expenditure which will now include **an additional $70 billion** of more government administrative workers in the IRS and other agencies to just administer the Affordable Care Act. Add to that the billions of dollars spent by insurance carriers and providers just to deal with bureaucratic paperwork issues. Then, add to that the billions of dollars asked to support medical care which includes all the Medicaid programs as well as all the annual insurance premiums paid into the insurance companies. Only a dramatic rescue plan can produce the needed result.

The Carpathia Health Plan is the solution because it revises the roles of all parties involved. The total sum game cuts the costs to all citizens in half. Taxes will be able to be substantially reduced. Although this may sound unrealistic, please appreciate the impact that this plan will have on the delivery of healthcare across this country.

Nothing described thus far should initially apply to Medicare which remains outside of this system at least until the system is proven successful and all the bugs worked out. Medicare and all Medicare recipients are therefore excluded.

The Carpathia Health Plan replaces Medicaid and saves the billions of dollars that it pays for the inefficiencies in the Medicaid programs. Best of all, doctors will be happy to take care of the poor instead of refusing to accept Medicaid in so many cases.

With that as the backdrop, we can go forward to understand exactly how easy it will be to redirect those funds into a single, simple plan that will provide medical care for everyone by using the market system within the elective portion, thereby reducing the cost over the entire system. The layered bureaucracy that currently manages to fund all the acute and catastrophic care that is being provided at this very moment will more than fund this new plan. Therefore, no additional funding sources will actually be necessary to pay for the acute care portion of this program. Actuaries will substantiate this statement. Let's look at how this plan can be funded in a very transparent and simple fashion.

Chapter 13: Two Pools to Fund Healthcare

Essentially there are two pools of funds. They are divided along the lines of the definitions previously discussed. Each pool is funded slightly differently. If the provider is providing urgent care, he bills one central fund which represents the pool of monies from several sources. He bills the fees that he has posted for the procedures that he has described. He can bill no more or no less. When he performs a service defined within the catastrophic definition, he bills the same posted fee to the catastrophic fund and does not collect the co-pay from the patient.

Carpathia Health Plan Provides For <u>All</u> Health Needs

Two Pools of Funds

**All Health Care is Paid for
From One of These Two Pools**

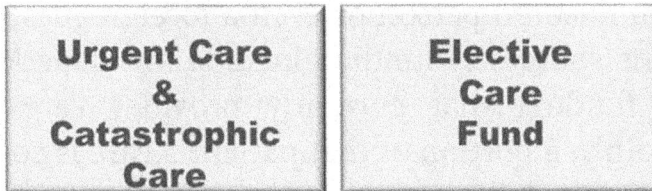

Urgent Care & Catastrophic Care	Elective Care Fund

When the patient receives care defined as catastrophic or urgent care, no second opinion threshold applies and they certainly won't be asked to pay any co-pay. The funding derives as follows:

How is the Urgent/Catastrophic Pool Funded?

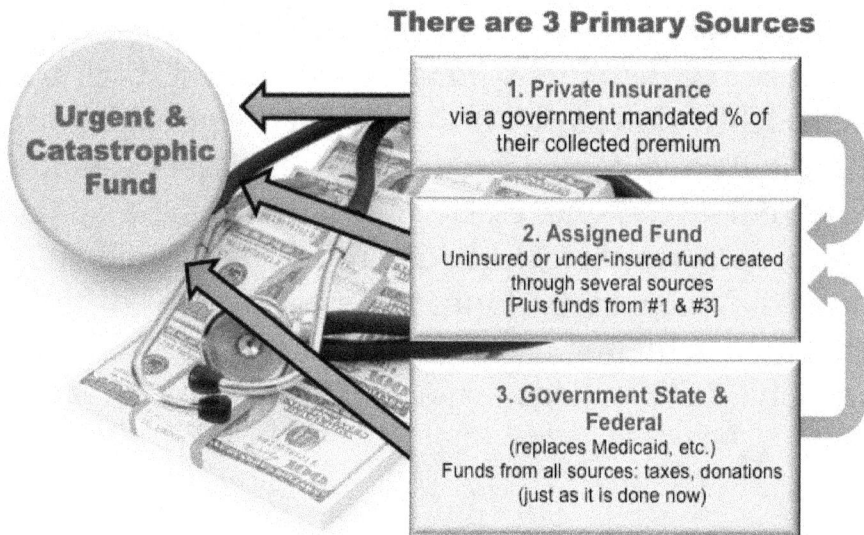

There are 3 Primary Sources

Urgent & Catastrophic Fund

1. Private Insurance
via a government mandated % of their collected premium

2. Assigned Fund
Uninsured or under-insured fund created through several sources
[Plus funds from #1 & #3]

3. Government State & Federal
(replaces Medicaid, etc.)
Funds from all sources: taxes, donations (just as it is done now)

The funding sources for urgent care are actually very similar to the way that urgent care is funded today. These funds are currently more than adequate.

Today, if an uninsured person or even a foreign guest gets hit by a truck, the sources of funding include the same Medicaid government funding that currently provides care to that patient. Certainly, a portion of that patient's care is covered by the hospital's overbilling of many private patients, which unfortunately creates even more distortion of who's paying for what. Private premiums even now pay part of the care for the uninsured.

The previous diagram simply spells this out very clearly. The annual invoices for private insurance premiums will, quite transparently, spell it out even better, as illustrated below:

How are Private Insurance Premiums Calculated by Companies?

Each company is notified annually by the government as to how much is required of their premium dollar to help fund the:

1. **Uninsured or underinsured fund (x% of premium)**
2. **UC Fund (x% of premium)**

These %s will vary annually but will be the same for all insurance companies

Insurance bill to each insured looks like this

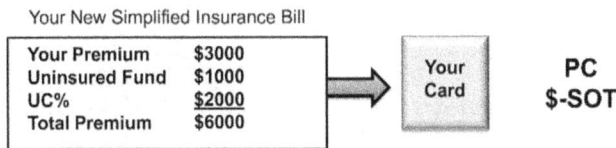

Your New Simplified Insurance Bill

Your Premium	$3000
Uninsured Fund	$1000
UC%	$2000
Total Premium	$6000

Your Card → PC $-SOT

If you look at this insurance premium invoice statement you will see only three line items. This is the ultimate in transparency.

Each insurance company will be advised at the beginning of each year by the government actuaries, how much of the **uninsured burden** the private sector will be asked to cover. Their company will have to bear a proportional amount of the total. In a similar fashion, the government actuaries will inform the private sector as to how much they will have to bear to cover the **urgent care/catastrophic fund**. Each private company will be assessed proportionally.

Each insurance company will then divide that amount up over the number of their insureds and that figure will be printed on your monthly invoice. Funding does not get more transparent than that!

These government assessments will be distributed evenly across all the private insurance companies and will be the total contribution needed to fund those specific pools after all government funds have already been absorbed within those categories.

The individual's insurance premium statement will clearly itemize that portion of the total premium that has been assigned to them via the two government pools, as well the amount that they are actually paying for the type of insurance that they had selected. That portion will depend on the specific percent co-pay "PC" and "SOT" that the individual selected. This will be described in later chapters.

It is important to appreciate that the Urgent Care Fund will completely and fully cover the privately insured consumers in the exact same way that it covers the urgent care of the poor, underinsured and uninsured. Not by what or who paid the premiums, but by the **definition. The private insurance companies are completely free of those costs for their insured.** If a person who is covered by private insurance gets hit by a truck or has a serious illness, the catastrophic fund covers the entire cost of care. The private companies have prepaid for the urgent care of their insureds via the urgent care percentage assessment, transparently identified on their premium bill.

Chapter 14: Options to Fund Elective Care

There are only two variables to keep in mind when a person obtains insurance coverage for elective care: the percent co-pay and the second opinion threshold (SOT). Private insurance can be purchased on the Internet. The insurance companies will compete, but each is free to charge whatever premium they wish based on just these two variables. The consumer will make the final decision as to what he or she wishes to purchase and how much they wish to pay.

In a similar way, depending on income, anyone can purchase or be assigned government-sponsored coverage based on the same two variables. The person's accompanying card simply provides the basic information to the provider and represents the criteria of the two variables that apply to any given patient.

It is that simple.

How is the Elective Pool Funded?

There are 3 Primary Sources

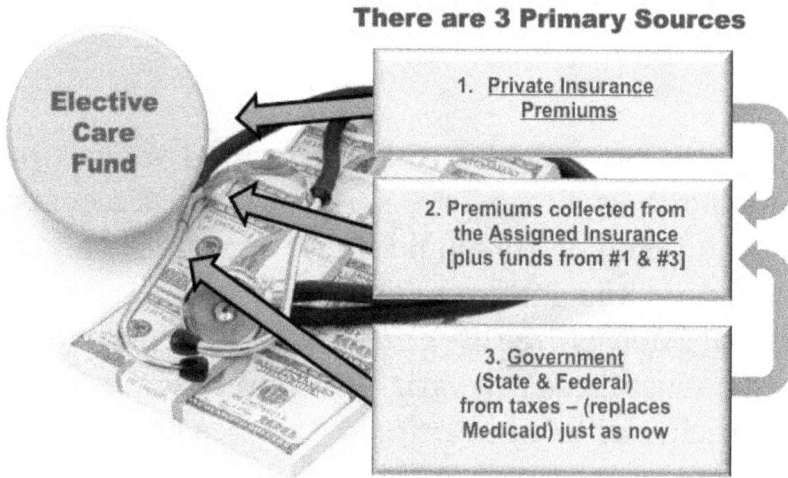

Elective Care Fund

1. Private Insurance Premiums

2. Premiums collected from the Assigned Insurance [plus funds from #1 & #3]

3. Government (State & Federal) from taxes – (replaces Medicaid) just as now

When providers offer treatment that is defined as elective care they bill their posted fee to either the insurance company or to the elective care fund. They must bill the patient the percent co-pay described on the patient's insurance card. The amount that the provider bills the fund or the insurance carrier is of course minus whatever he or she collected from the patient. The physician is obligated to collect the percent co-pay from the patient. The patient's insurance card (which is to be used only for elective care) will simply describe the three key pieces of information required by the provider:

1. The name and address of the payor (insurance company or elective care fund) on the back of the insurance card.

2. The percent co-pay - front of insurance card.

3. The second opinion threshold (SOT) – front of insurance card.

Every person can obtain an insurance card which will provide him with access to elective care! The next question that needs to be answered is: how does a person obtain an insurance card? There are three options:

Option 1:

Purchase insurance from the government-managed insurance website.

Can Everyone Obtain a Healthcare Card?
There are Three Options!
Option #1
Private Insurance Card

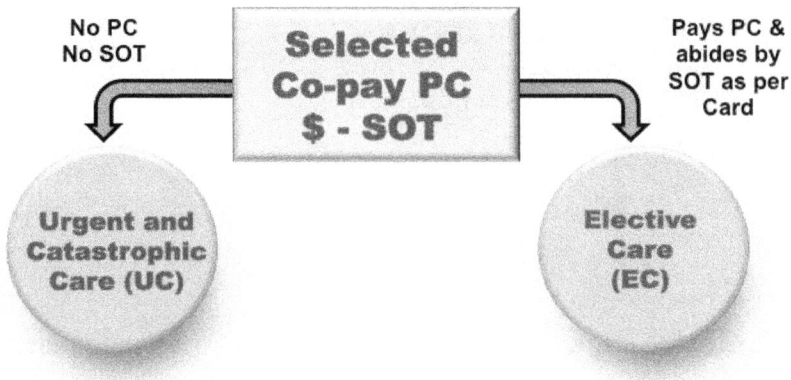

No PC
No SOT

Selected Co-pay PC $ - SOT

Pays PC & abides by SOT as per Card

Urgent and Catastrophic Care (UC)

Elective Care (EC)

Option 2:

For low-income individuals—a means-tested card from their hospital outreach clinic.

Can Everyone Obtain a Healthcare Card?
There are Three Options!

Option #2
Means Tested Card

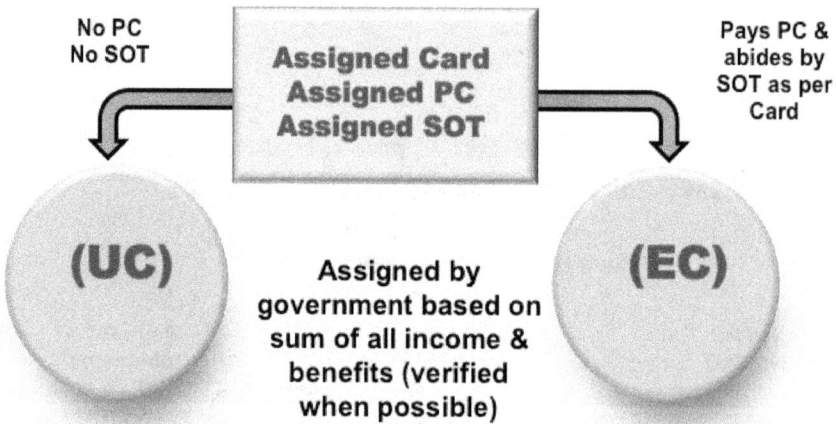

No PC
No SOT

Pays PC &
abides by
SOT as per
Card

Assigned Card
Assigned PC
Assigned SOT

(UC)

(EC)

Assigned by
government based on
sum of all income &
benefits (verified
when possible)

Option 3:

An individual decides not to select either option #1 or #2.

The next plausible question would be: What if you had no insurance card? To fully understand the implications of that question please keep in mind that the free market competition will have lowered the providers' fees to real or actual market value. This means that the posted fees will no longer be astronomical but rather realistic and balanced by the competition and the real costs, giving providers fair profit with minimal overhead.

Can Everyone Obtain a Healthcare Card?
There are Three Options!
Option #3

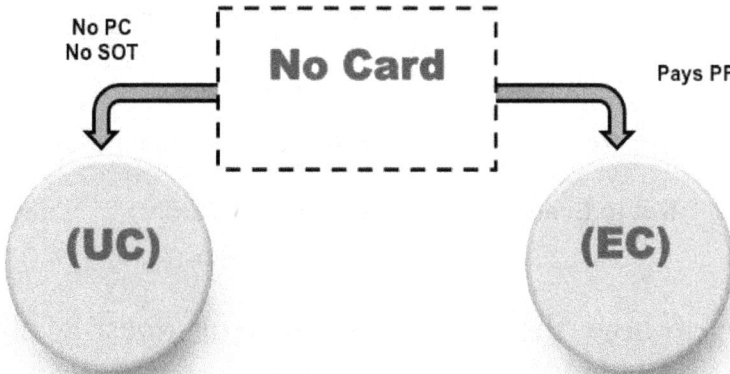

No PC
No SOT

No Card

Pays PF

(UC)

(EC)

However, even if an individual chooses not to select any of the options, they will still be able to fully access both urgent and elective care at low and realistic fees brought down to actual market value because of the Carpathia Health Plan.

And What if You Have No Card?
How Would You Access Elective Care?

Option #3

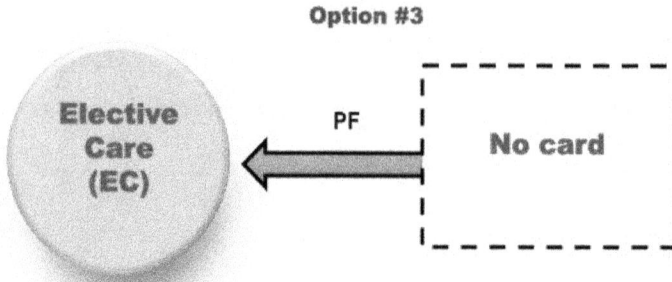

Rich or Poor, You Can Choose Not to Purchase Insurance
OR
Not to Even Apply for an Assigned Card

Irrespective of how the consumer does or doesn't obtain coverage, the providers' fees would be transparent and available for all to see and providers would not be permitted to charge more than that fee.

> **Summary:** Elective care is billed to the insurer minus the percent co-pay in Option #1, and in Option #2, from the uninsured fund, according to the rules. In Option #3, the full provider fee would be billed to the patient who chose not to obtain any insurance.

> Despite the pathway, the Carpathia Health Plan lowers fees across all options and permits full access for everyone. Urgent care is available for all members of society, and even those with no insurance card are fully served because all such bills for urgent care are billed directly to the urgent care fund.

Regardless of which of the three options are used to obtain an insurance card for elective care, there are no restrictions on what care you can seek. In addition, since there are no provider networks, there are no restrictions on the providers that you can seek. Finally, there are no denials, penalties, deductibles, necessary referrals, or bureaucratic algorithms that will affect your access to elective medical care.

It was previously stated that one of the key government responsibilities was to create an actuarial curve to provide for a means-tested insurance card and access to hospital outreach clinics to guarantee that care will be provided to all members of society.

Does everyone have to buy insurance?

Are there penalties to the individual or employer if you choose not to buy insurance?

The answer to these two questions is an absolute. and unequivocal, "No!!"

How Elective Care is Paid For

With Insurance

Who Does The Provider Bill?
What Does the Provider Charge?

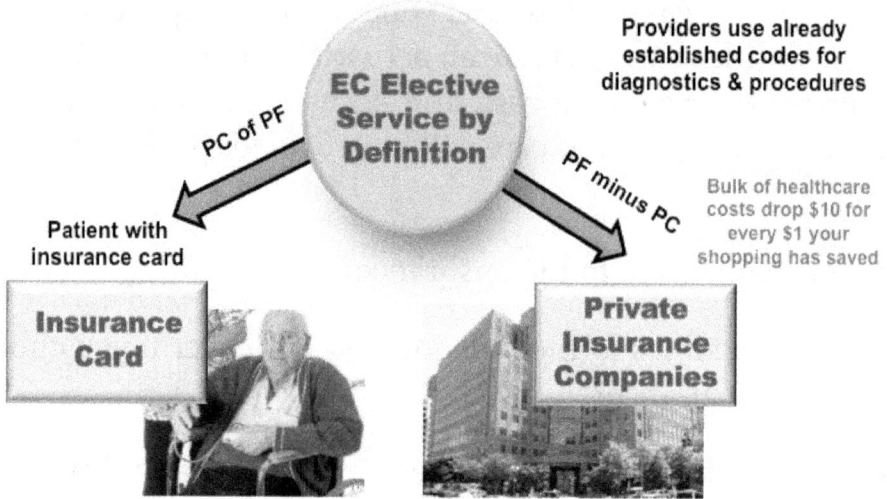

Providers use already established codes for diagnostics & procedures

EC Elective Service by Definition

PC of PF

PF minus PC

Bulk of healthcare costs drop $10 for every $1 your shopping has saved

Patient with insurance card

Insurance Card

Private Insurance Companies

How Elective Care is Paid For
Without Insurance

Low income or no income patients are provided with a means-tested insurance card provided by the Government at a hospital intake desk.

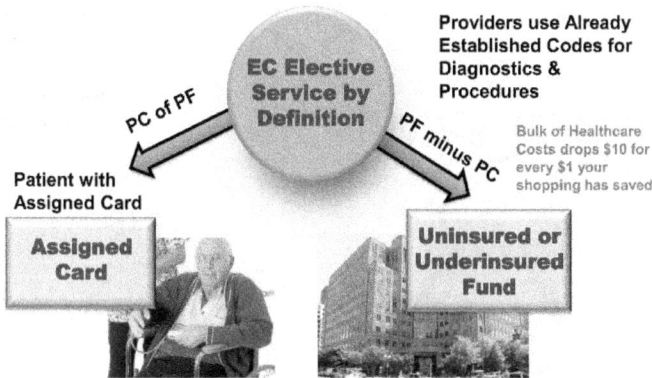

Who Does The Provider Bill?
& What Does the Provider Charge?

EC Elective Service by Definition

PC of PF

PF minus PC

Providers use Already Established Codes for Diagnostics & Procedures

Bulk of Healthcare Costs drops $10 for every $1 your shopping has saved

Patient with Assigned Card

Assigned Card

Uninsured or Underinsured Fund

How Elective Care is Paid For
With No Insurance Card

(Patient has no insurance and no insurance card but wishes ELECTIVE CARE.)

Who Does The Provider Bill?
& What Does the Provider Charge?

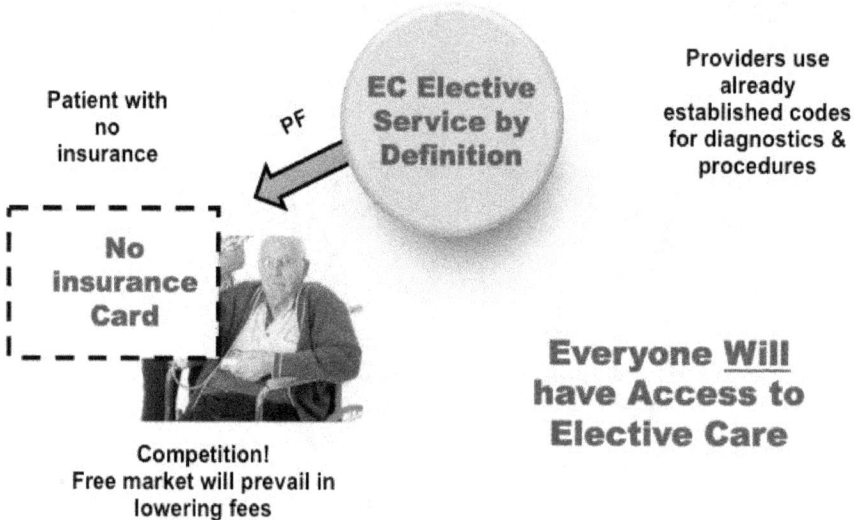

Patient with no insurance

PF

EC Elective Service by Definition

Providers use already established codes for diagnostics & procedures

No insurance Card

Everyone **Will** have Access to Elective Care

Competition! Free market will prevail in lowering fees

Where Do Patients Access Elective Care?

Elective Care	ER Triage nurse applies definitions for treatment for admission or treatment.
Doctors' Offices	
Hospital Outreach Clinics	(Only UC is to be treated in ERs.)
Drug Stores	ER providers must send patients who
Hospitals	require only EC to Hospital Outreach
Surgicenters	Clinics or Private Doctors
Etc.	

What can these providers charge?
ONLY THEIR POSTED FEES
Free Market Will Work Over Short Time

If a patient goes to the emergency room for the first time with a non-urgent issue such as a cold, once the triage nurse or physician affirms that the patient is not suffering from a life-threatening condition, they are required to refer the patient to the hospital outreach clinic the following day, in the exact same way they would refer a patient to a private physician. This is not different than before, but the new definitions prohibit the ER physician from beginning to treat any patient suffering from a non-urgent condition.

When the patient appears in the emergency room for a second time with the same non-urgent condition they would have already been given a means-tested insurance card at the same ER intake desk, and this time referred directly to the hospital outreach clinic. These new definitions will ultimately, reduce the inappropriate use of the emergency room by the uninsured, or even by insured patients. Again, the system will experience a marked cost reduction.

Chapter 15: Accessing Urgent Care

Finally, free health care for all and the funding mechanism to support it!

This plan establishes a transparent funding structure that provides for free care for the entire population for any and all treatments related to any and all life- or limb-threatening care, i.e. URGENT CARE (non-elective by definition). No longer will there be cases of an impoverished mother unable to purchase insulin for her diabetic daughter. No longer will we question how the medical care is provided for an impoverished soul who gets hit by a truck.

Please recall, we previously discussed that when care is provided for life-threatening or limb-threatening defined conditions, the provider of that care still must bill only what he or she posted as the accepted fee and cannot bill the patient for any co-pay, nor is the patient bound to their insurance contract to obtain second opinions (which may be required for elective care).

The proper billing path is decided when the diagnosis is made. Currently no patient is treated without a diagnosis being attached to the billing invoice. No procedure is billed without a CPT code. All medical billing already requires each diagnosis be submitted with a procedure code. This new concept does not change the current procedure code requirement in any way.

Patients initially access emergency care in a hospital or urgent care setting. (No different than what is done currently.)

Sometimes patients are told that they might have a life-threatening condition in the doctor's office.

No matter where such a diagnosis is made, a life- or limb-threatening condition is paid for via the appropriate funded pool for as long as the patient is being treated for that particular condition. It is important to add that in the current system of medical coding the diagnosis is already tied to the various procedures appropriate for treatment of that specific diagnosis. This already functioning apparatus remains intact and will be fully utilized in the Carpathia Health Plan.

Can Everyone Access Urgent/ Catastrophic Care? Yes! Everyone Rich & Poor

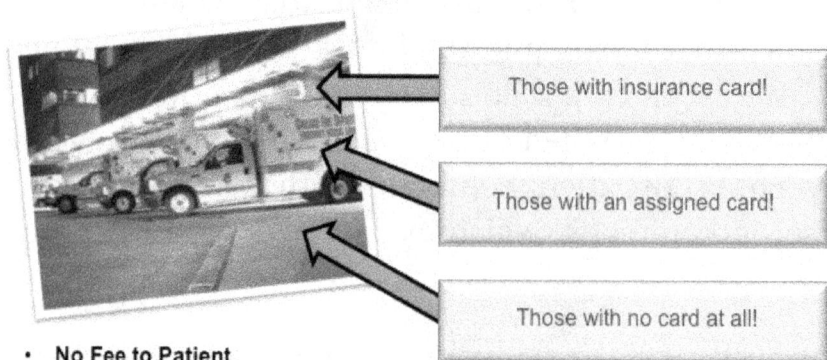

Those with insurance card!

Those with an assigned card!

Those with no card at all!

- No Fee to Patient
- No % Co-pay PC
- No SOT
- Everyone has a right to any care that is life-threatening or limb-threatening as defined by the accepted definitions.

There will be no change in the location or manner in which a patient receives urgent care.

Where Do Patients Access Elective Care?

Elective Care Doctors' Offices Hospital Outreach Clinics Drug Stores Hospitals Surgicenters Etc.	ER Triage nurse applies definitions for treatment for admission or treatment. (Only UC is to be treated in ERs.) ER providers must send patients who require only EC to Hospital Outreach Clinics or Private Doctors

What can these providers charge?
ONLY THEIR POSTED FEES
Free Market Will Work Over Short Time

All urgent care is billed directly to the urgent care fund. It is important to note that any attempts to misleadingly categorize certain treatments as urgent (which could be a source of fraud and abuse) would be quickly and easily nipped in the bud because all the bills are sent to a single central office and can easily be monitored and addressed at that point. Also, a fee that is greater than two standards of deviation greater than the mean will produce an alert in the system. Investigation and prosecution of appropriate cases of fraud would be identified at this early juncture.

Who Does the Provider Bill?
What Does the Provider Charge?

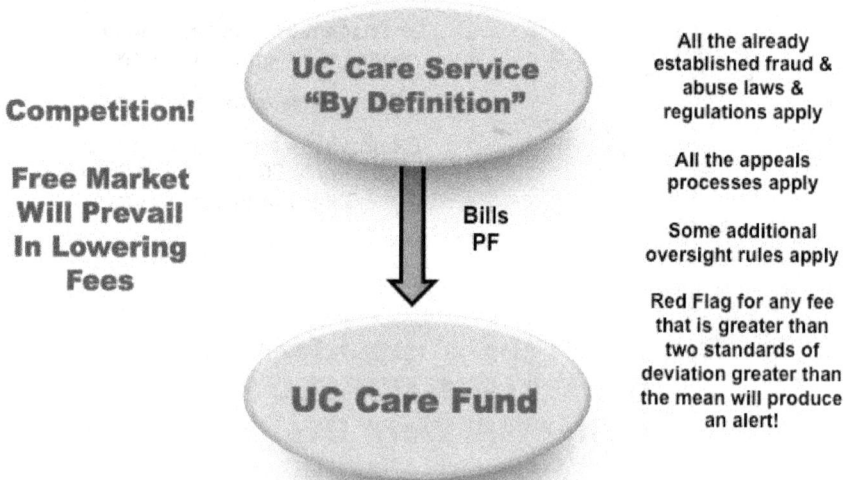

Competition!

**Free Market
Will Prevail
In Lowering
Fees**

UC Care Service
"By Definition"

Bills
PF

UC Care Fund

All the already
established fraud &
abuse laws &
regulations apply

All the appeals
processes apply

Some additional
oversight rules apply

Red Flag for any fee
that is greater than
two standards of
deviation greater than
the mean will produce
an alert!

In this way, the best possible treatment, equal for all, both the rich and the poor, is fully available to our entire society; with or without insurance cards, with or without insurance, with or without even a means-tested card.

Recap from previous chapters:

Examples of life-threatening and limb-threatening care:

- Catastrophic care
- Cancer care
- Acute cardiac care, including cardiac catheterization, stents, angioplasties, acute pulmonary care
- Fracture care
- Anything that threatens life or limb either in the short-term or long-term or anything, the treatment of which if delayed, might jeopardize life or limb

How is the Urgent/Catastrophic Pool Funded?

There are 3 Primary Sources

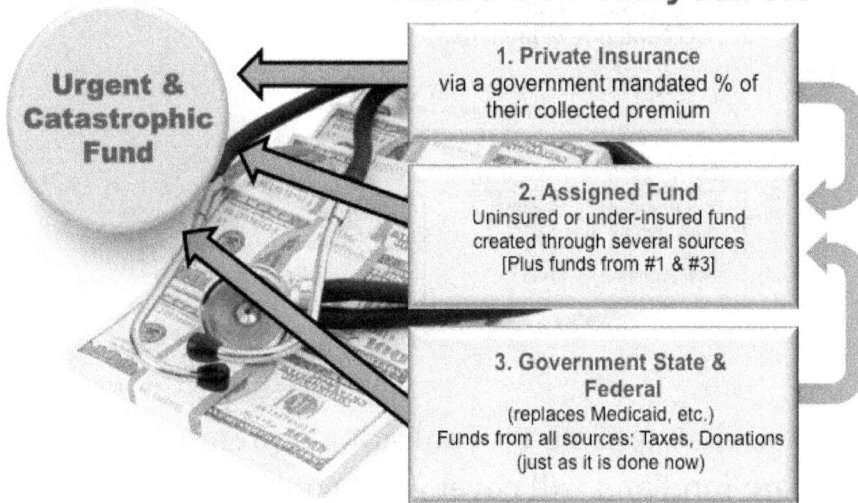

Urgent & Catastrophic Fund

1. Private Insurance
via a government mandated % of their collected premium

2. Assigned Fund
Uninsured or under-insured fund created through several sources
[Plus funds from #1 & #3]

3. Government State & Federal
(replaces Medicaid, etc.)
Funds from all sources: Taxes, Donations
(just as it is done now)

The Carpathia Health Plan replaces Medicaid in all states. Most funds previously designated for Medicaid will be diverted to fund the uninsured or underinsured fund, and a portion will be directed to the catastrophic fund in the same proportion as the actuaries designate for all other insurers.

How are Private Insurance Premiums Calculated by Companies?

Each company is notified annually by the government as to how much is required of their premium dollar to help fund the:

1. **Uninsured or underinsured fund (x% of premium)**
2. **UC Fund (x% of premium)**

These %s will vary annually but will be the same for all insurance companies

Insurance bill to each insured looks like this

Your New Simplified Insurance Bill

Your Premium	$3000
Uninsured Fund	$1000
UC%	$2000
Total Premium	$6000

➡ Your Card

PC
$-SOT

The $2,000 that appears on your annual premium went to the urgent care fund and will cover all of your urgent care.

Chapter 16: Review and Further Details

1. All patients have skin in the game for all elective care.

2. All urgent care is free to the rich and poor.

3. Anyone can go to any willing licensed provider in any state (no networks).

4. Providers get their full fee and competition will control prices.

5. Paperwork, bureaucracy, and administrative costs will be minimized.

6. Government has an appropriate role (not too big or too small).

7. Fraud and abuse will be punished severely (central locations receive all bills).

8. The SOT replaces billions of dollars of bureaucracy. (Second opinions for EC is beneficial and doesn't hurt anyone. It better informs us all).

9. Patients can shop quality and cost as easily as they can shop for a TV. The mystery veil is removed. The separation of cost from care is removed as it applies to elective care.

10. Patients shop for providers and insurance the same way.

Everything that has been discussed to this point was specifically and exclusively silent on some key issues:

1. All insurances can be sold across state lines. There are no networks. Any patient/consumer can go to

any "willing provider" in any state.

2. There are no pre-existing conditions mentioned because in this plan there are no pre-existing conditions that would affect a patient's/consumer's ability to purchase insurance. This is purposely not mentioned because, as you will see, pre-existing conditions have no place in, nor are even considered in the pricing of insurance premiums. The issue of pre-existing conditions is addressed at the time insurance is purchased for each individual. If you have a pre-existing condition that causes you to anticipate a lot of upcoming care, you would search for a policy with a low co-pay and a slightly higher SOT. You would pay more upfront but in the end, the difference will be slight. This would end the fright over pre-existing conditions.

3. Children (of the age of 26 and even beyond) remaining at home with their parents can be added to their parents' insurance contract.

4. There are no employer mandates or penalties imposed upon the individual or the employer (there doesn't need to be in a free market system).

5. There are no individual subsidies needed, or extra and hidden taxes in this system (there doesn't need to be any in a competitive market system).

6. No need to hire thousands of additional administrators or create new government departments. Forget the $70 billion estimated and new bureaucratic costs that provide no medical benefit to any person recently announced to implement the Affordable Care Act.

7. No need to expand the IRS to collect any new taxes.

8. Medical savings plans will be expanded and are part of the Carpathia Health Plan.

9. There are no rationing committees.

10. There is no need to grant waivers to special groups.

Chapter 17: Behind the Scenes

Actuaries Are Hard at Work

Carpathia Health Plan
Behind The Scenes
How Does It Really Work?

Here is how it really works. This complex chapter will be presented in the order that best addresses the questions that have arisen by now. The reader is asked to suspend the requirement for full comprehension until after all the unique aspects of the program have been reviewed and all the pieces of the puzzle are re-assembled.

Both at the insurance companies and in Washington, actuarial expertise is required to make sure appropriate funding is provided and directed in the correct manner.

The calculations under the Carpathia Health Plan will be much simpler than they are today and based on dramatically different parameters. There are only two parameters to be measured. These come down to a simple curve on a graph based on actuarial fundamentals. Your full attention will be needed here to understand the simplicity of this new concept.

The only two variables that have to be calculated and that go on an insurance card are the PC and SOT.

How Do Insurance Companies and Government Means Tested Formulas Set the Only Two Variables in the System?

Through PC & SOT (The same way they do now, by targeting their markets and using actual calculations).

How do insurance companies determine their premiums?

Behind the scenes, actuaries are hard at work.

First, they determine the premium that would be related to the percent co-pay they wish to offer their customers, as shown below:

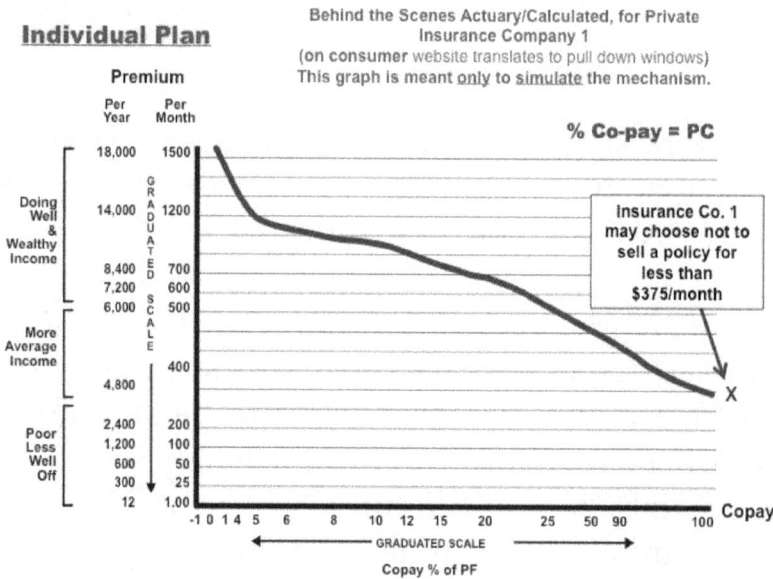

The higher the premium that the consumer chooses, the lower the percent co-pay and vice versa; the lower the percent co-pay is chosen by the consumer, the higher the premium.

Then they would figure out the second opinion threshold (SOT) that they wish to offer their customers for a given premium. As below:

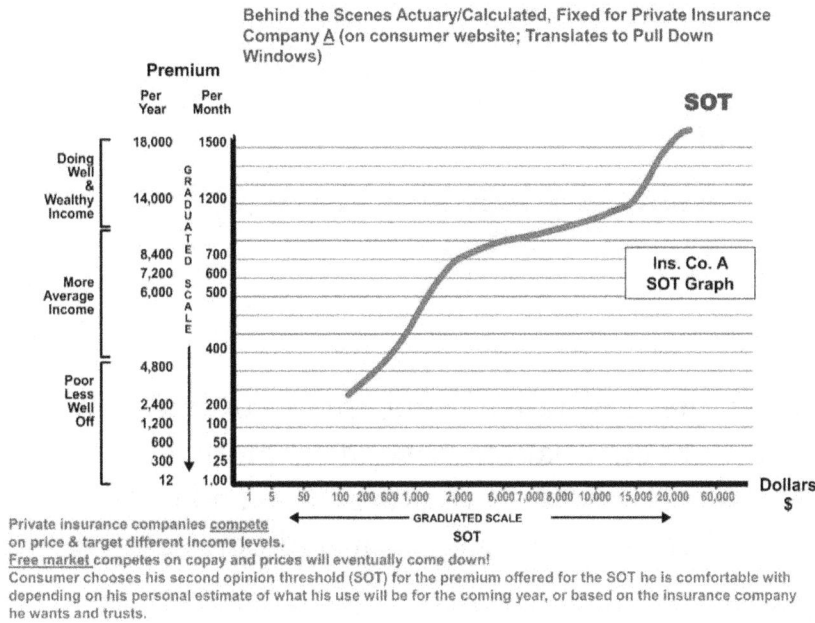

Behind the Scenes Actuary/Calculated, Fixed for Private Insurance Company A (on consumer website; Translates to Pull Down Windows)

Private insurance companies compete on price & target different income levels.
Free market competes on copay and prices will eventually come down!
Consumer chooses his second opinion threshold (SOT) for the premium offered for the SOT he is comfortable with depending on his personal estimate of what his use will be for the coming year, or based on the insurance company he wants and trusts.

The higher the premium that the consumer chooses, the higher the threshold (high SOT) that requires a second opinion and vice versa; the lower the threshold is that triggers the need for a second opinion (low SOT) the lower the premium.

The process requires that each insurance company targets their potential customers by income level and where they wish to be in the marketplace. Insurance Company A's graph might look like this:

Behind the Scenes Actuary/Calculated, Fixed for Private Insurance
Combination of Each Company's PC and SOT (consumer website;
will see this as pull down windows). Insurance Company A
Target Market $600 per month Premium

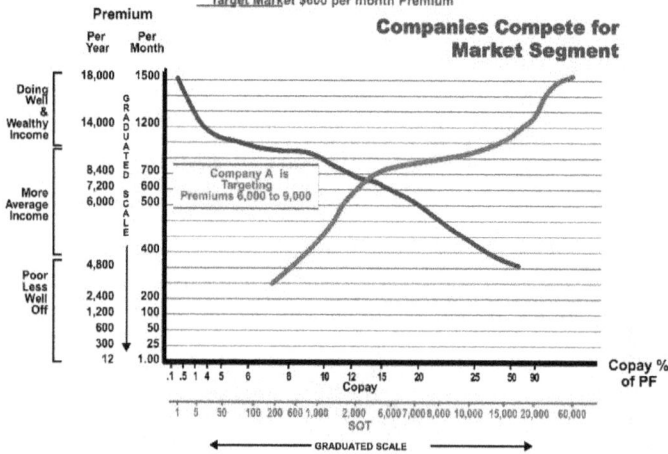

Companies Compete for Market Segment

Premium
Per Year — Per Month

GRADUATED SCALE

Doing Well & Wealthy Income	18,000	1500
	14,000	1200
	8,400	700
More Average Income	7,200	600
	6,000	500
	4,800	400
Poor Less Well Off	2,400	200
	1,200	100
	600	50
	300	25
	12	1.00

Company A Is Targeting Premiums 6,000 to 9,000

Copay: .1 .5 1 4 5   6   8   10 12 15   20   25 50 90

Copay % of PF

SOT: 1 5 90 100 200 600 1,900 2,000 6,000 7,000 8,000 10,000 15,000 20,000 60,000

GRADUATED SCALE

This simply means that Insurance Company A considers their ideal market, households that earn slightly more than the average income and can afford a premium of $6,000 to $9,000 per year, and would consider a policy that had between a 10% to 20% co-pay.

They also calculated that their target market would be interested in a SOT range between $1,800 and $6,000. The premium that they would charge for those two variables that a customer may select would come right from this simple two-parameter, actuarially-generated chart, specifically designed for and by Insurance Company A to capture a specific portion of the private insurance market.

Insurance Company A would then convert this graph to drop-down windows on a simple website that would compete with other insurance carriers for the same or different segments of the market. The entire insurance industry would thereby become simplified, totally transparent, almost bureaucratically weightless, no longer in control of your healthcare, no longer between you and your physician, and fully competitive in the marketplace. Finally, health insurance would be what it is in every other industry: not in control of your life.

Meanwhile, Insurance Company B may target households with incomes that were willing to pay between $5,000 and $7,000 per year and accept % co-pay of 12-to-15% and an SOT of $2,000-to-$4,000.

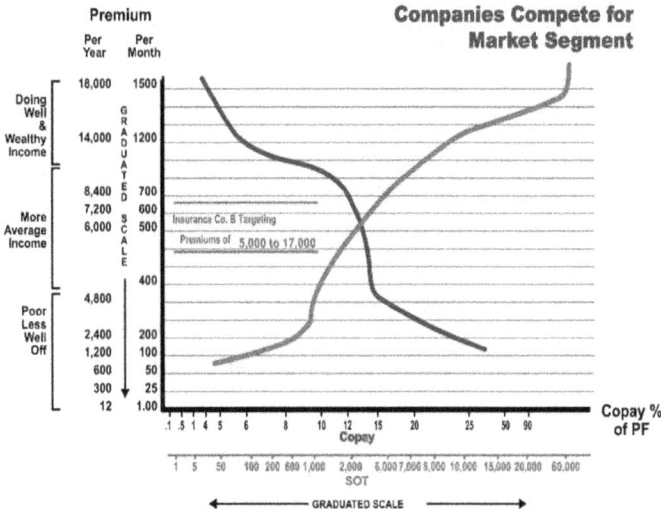

Individual Plan

Behind the Scenes Actuary/Calculated, Fixed for Private Insurance Combination of Each Company's PC and SOT (consumer website; will see this as pull down windows) Comparing Insurance Company B Target Market $520 per month Premium

Companies Compete for Market Segment

Other insurance companies would produce similar graphs that may appear like this behind the scenes:

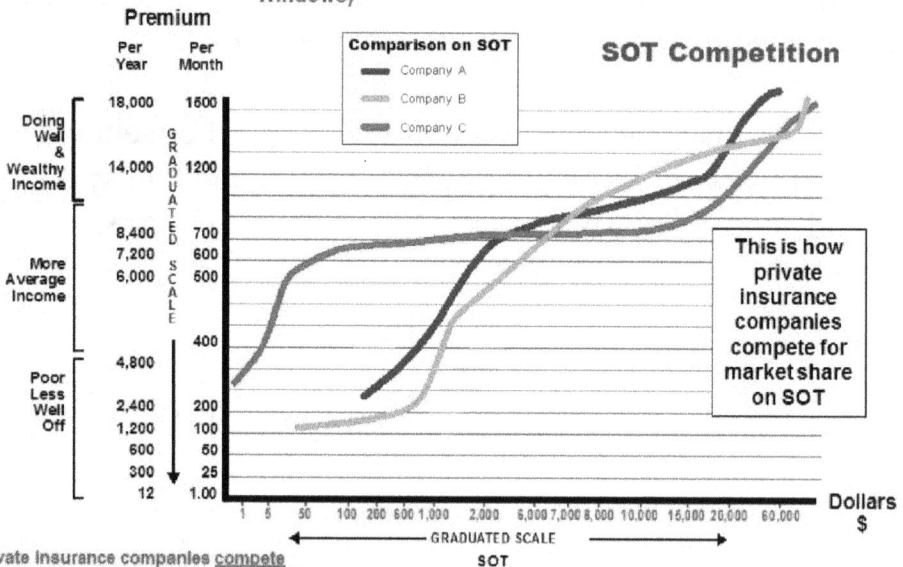

Individual Plan

Behind the Scenes Actuary/Calculated, Fixed for Private Insurance Companies (on consumer website; Translates to Pull Down Windows)

Premium

	Per Year	Per Month
	18,000	1600
Doing Well & Wealthy Income	14,000	1200
	8,400	700
	7,200	600
More Average Income	6,000	500
		400
	4,800	
Poor Less Well Off	2,400	200
	1,200	100
	600	50
	300	25
	12	1.00

GRADUATED SCALE

Comparison on SOT
Company A
Company B
Company C

SOT Competition

This is how private insurance companies compete for market share on SOT

1   5   50   100 200 600 1,000   2,000   6,000 7,000 8,000 10,000 15,000 20,000   60,000

Dollars $

GRADUATED SCALE
SOT

Private insurance companies compete on price & target different income levels.
Free market competes on copay and prices will eventually come down!
Consumer chooses his second opinion threshold (SOT) for the premium offered for the SOT he is comfortable with depending on his personal estimate of what his use will be for the coming year, or based on the insurance company he wants and trusts.

Pre-existing conditions are now conditions for which the individual decides and makes his own choices. The shape and slope of these curves presented by each of the insurance carriers competing for their market share represent the total picture of the premiums being offered to the consumer. It is not any more complicated than that! The carriers will compete in an open and transparent marketplace.

The webpage representation where the insurance companies actually compete in the marketplace would be presented to the public as no more than drop down box/user-friendly conversion of the underlying actuary curves produced and would look like this to the consumer purchasing insurance:

Robert Dennis, MD

User Friendly Window for Consumer Insurance.
How Do Patients Select Insurance?

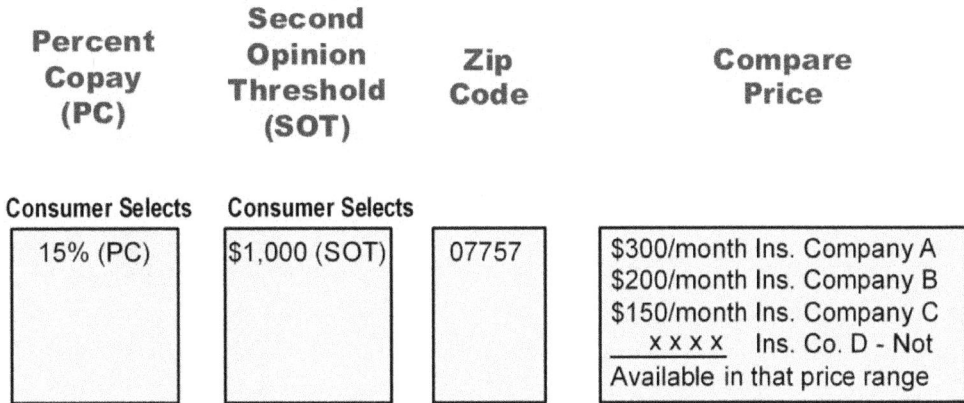

Percent Copay (PC)	Second Opinion Threshold (SOT)	Zip Code	Compare Price
Consumer Selects	Consumer Selects		
15% (PC)	$1,000 (SOT)	07757	$300/month Ins. Company A $200/month Ins. Company B $150/month Ins. Company C x x x x Ins. Co. D - Not Available in that price range

A patient with severe medical problems and pre-existing conditions would probably select a low percent co-pay and a high SOT. **If those conditions were already diagnosed as life and/or limb threatening, none of this would matter, as all such care would be FREE.**

It is **most important** to keep in mind that with the Carpathia Health Plan, insurance is only for elective care. Pre-existing, urgent medical conditions are covered by all of us. For all of us, insurance would only be for elective care.

(Full Disclaimer: These graphs and estimates are just that—rough estimates provided in order to give the reader an idea as to how this plan actually operates behind the scenes. We do not claim to be actuaries and these numbers and data are fictitious and for illustrative purposes only.)

Chapter 18: The Government's Role

A Free-Market System

Government actuaries provide insurance cards for elective care to patients who cannot afford private insurance, or can afford private insurance but choose the government plan instead for whatever reason.

The government plan is specifically designed to be very unattractive for wealthy households. Actuarial yet simple management of the slope of the curve is all that is required. The same graph, by its very design, provides a very fair and appropriate insurance plan for the uninsured or underinsured for elective care. It's no more complicated than that!

From this single simple curve (ZIP Code adjusted) and available at every hospital intake desk, low income households can be easily provided with insurance coverage for all elective care.

Assigned Care:

Behind the scenes actuaries are hard at work identifying income levels that qualify for specific assigned parameters of PC & SOT.

The Means Test sets up a simple and uniform mechanism to provide an assigned card to rich & poor alike.

> **Assigned Card**
> **% Copay $SOT**

Anyone and everyone is eligible for an assigned card if they so choose. The rich, the poor, and the newly welcomed visitors to our country can obtain a card. It is a pure function of their income. Income verification is required. Even if they make $2000 a year from picking fruit or mowing lawns and do not file taxes or if they make a poverty level income or millions of dollars, it doesn't matter. If they can show some proof of what their income is, either a high or low or zero, any and all of us will be able to obtain a government-issued assigned card.

Most of us who could afford insurance will find that the private market will charge us less and give us more than the assigned government card. But that is totally up to the individual. Yes, the government will compete with the private market but the private market will not want to target the low income brackets that the government program will be happy to cover. In this way, there can be no one without insurance for elective care unless they so choose. And again, we are all covered in full for all urgent care.

Please remember that this plan replaces Medicaid and all the funding that would normally be directed through the Medicaid program. All of that funding would now be redirected to this new plan—the assigned card program. The actuarial-designed government plan may look like this:

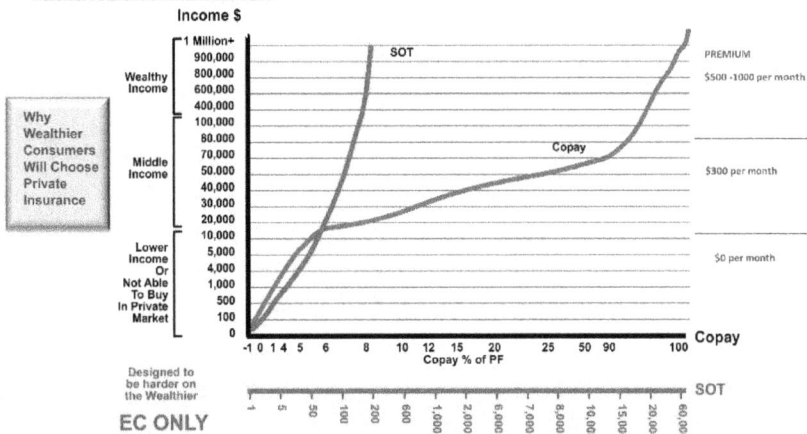

How Does The Government Go About Assigning A Card Based On Income?

By utilizing a simple, Actuary Generated Graph. This graph is uniform across the country and varies only by zip code.
This means test favors Lower Incomes but also permits anyone to apply.
The graph applies to both consumers who cannot afford private insurance and consumers who choose not to purchase private insurance.
The government cannot discriminate!

The graph below demonstrates why someone who could afford private insurance would not want the assigned plan. It would cause such a person to pay a higher co-pay and be required to go for more confirmatory second opinions than what a private plan would require for the same premium. The assigned plan is based solely on income, while the private insurance market is based on consumer choice. Again, this is limited to elective care only.

On the other hand, it would offer very low co-pays and reasonable second opinion requirements for low income households. Just by the shape of the curves and their slopes the entire system can be implemented and maintained easily.

The reader is reminded to recall that all of these graphs and cards apply exclusively to elective care and that the graphs are representations for illustrative purposes. The actual graph will be generated by actuarial calculations.

Assigned Plan

Behind the Scenes Actuary Calculated Graph. This is how simple it can be!
This graph is meant only to simulate the mechanism.

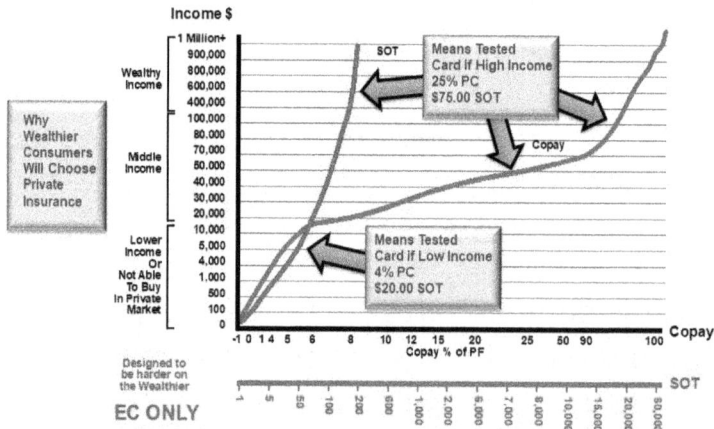

The government website to facilitate low income households in obtaining assigned insurance cards for elective care would look something like this:

Review Slide
How Does The Government
Apply a Universal Means Test?

**Go to Hospital &/or Hospital Outreach
Clinic Intake/Reception or Web Site**

Sum of All Sources of Income	Proof of Income	Zip	Sign Fraud Statement	Means PC	Means SOT
___ $___	___	___	"I affirm under	___	___
___ $___	___		penalty of the	___	___
___ $___	___		law..."	___	___
Total $___	___		Yes ___ No ___		

Who Can Apply for Assigned Insurance?
Anyone or Everyone
Means tested income will likely produce higher PC & lower
SOT than private carriers for wealthier

This user-friendly website will be accessed by anyone and also used by the hospital intake desk when they provide consumers with a means tested assigned insurance card.

Both the government and private insurance plans compete, but in very different demographic markets where private insurance would not want to be and where government insurance has to be because the funding is so very different.

Reminder: the website that insurance companies provide, you may recall, looks very similar, but the underlying curves used to generate these user-friendly websites are very different.

Chapter 19: Carpathia Health Plan and Specific Issues

How does the system handle chronic illness?

Some chronic but not urgent conditions:

- Adult onset diabetes
- Chronic heart problems
- Bipolar patients
- Thyroid patients
- Certain non-lethal tumor patients, etc.

By rewarding the patient directly for achieving certain goals, such as:

- Weight Loss
- Exercise
- Medication Compliance
- Accessing any form of preventative care or preventative testing

The plan acknowledges success with rewards programs similar to miles programs for credit cards.

The patients that improve their own state of health get immediate reduction in their co-pay and increase in their SOT.

How will the system handle huge hospital costs?

How can a normal patient afford to pay even his % co-pay (PC) of a huge hospital bill generated by an elective stay?

- Even though hospitals are Providers, they compete on the basis of their day-stay rates.
- Consumers can shop and select the most cost-effective hospital or surgicenter for elective procedures and workups.
- Most doctors work at several facilities (the patient has choices).
- Furthermore, additional hospital cost controls remain in place.
- And most importantly, the patient will only be responsible for a small percentage (perhaps 20%) of the patient's percent co-pay (PC) identified on the patient's insurance card.

(e.g.: Hospital bill for elective admission is $10,000. Patient has a 10% co-pay, 10% of 10,000=$1,000. But hospital can only bill patients 20% of their PC (20% of $1,000=$200).

How does the system handle routine check-ups and preventative care?

This is obviously elective care and subject to PC and SOT. However these fees are usually below the common SOT. These services can be shopped and "good behavior" will provide rewards (via PC reduction) directly to the patient via the "Rewards Program."

How does the system handle fraud and abuse?

How does the plan control for excessive fees for UC or for providers stretching the definition of UC for things that are not really urgent?

The same way we handle fraud & abuse and price fixing now: with severe penalties and investigation of red flags and alerts.

Also, if all the UC bills are going to the same place it will be much easier to identify the fraudulent behavior.

How does the plan handle cancer patients?

Very well! Cancer is usually life-threatening. Therefore, all patients with an established cancer diagnosis fall under the definition of UC. They are not required to pay their PC nor obligated to abide by their SOT.

However, the workup needed to arrive at the cancer diagnosis does come under the definition of elective care.

Cancer workup = Elective Care

Cancer treatment = Urgent or Catastrophic

Other Controversial Issues:

After appropriate laws are complied with, the specialty committees along with government will define which diagnoses are elective and which are not.

Chapter 20: **Summation**

This concept is by no means fully packaged. It requires further input by other experts, and from all six players. The country's healthcare is vital to all of us. It should not be imposed upon us, but rather each of us needs to participate in the process and make it better. Inputs from all sectors and all participants are vital at this juncture so that the final outcome, with full appreciation for how painful change can be, will be the best it can be and far better than any other country's healthcare program.

There is a temptation to compare our country to others. This is simply not valid when it comes to healthcare. Just because other developed countries have universal healthcare does not mean you can extract that one piece of another society and culture, and transplant it here unless you look at all the other components of that society and adopt them as well. This includes legal environments as well.

We are a unique country and one size does not fit all. For example, other societies are not burdened with the same malpractice litigation concerns as are we. Therefore, if we adopt, for instance, Norway's health system we must also adopt their legal system. Actually, we can and should do better than has ever been done elsewhere rather than aim at mimicking another country's flawed plan. That is not good enough.

The U.S. can and will set the bar higher, by example, than other countries. The world will mimic us as it relates to quality, availability and access when we implement the Carpathia Health Plan. We will not only be able to rescue survivors but also save the ship from sinking in the first place.

SUMMARY

1. When and if this new paradigm or parts of it ever become part of a new guideline is, of course, conjecture.
2. However, with some tweaking and expansion, it might reach 500 pages of simplicity, which is far better than 2500-3000 pages of needless complication that is currently layered in our current health delivery plans.

Key
Characteristics of
The Carpathia Health
Plan

- Easy to understand and implement

- **Enhances patient's choice** and the doctor/patient relationship

- Assumes that both **rich and poor are equally able to make informed healthcare decisions** (in the same way that we decide which TV, food, or appliance to purchase – **value vs. price (we are good at this)**

- Relies on **legitimate second opinions** instead of: rationing committees, government penalties, subsidies, referrals, authorizations, provider networks, deductibles and bureaucratic obstructions, etc.

Appendix: Executive Summary

Carpathia Health Plan

Major points only – Please see more information at www.CarpathiaHealthPlan.com

A.   Providers: Post all fees and qualifications

B.   Health Insurance Companies:

    1.   Contribute to two pools:

        a.   Uninsured pool

        b.   Catastrophic pool

    2.   Pay providers posted fees

    3.   Sell plans that vary only by co-pay amounts and the threshold amounts required for mandatory second opinions

    4.   Encourage savings plans

    5.   Portable state-to-state plans

    6.   No pre-existing illness clauses

    7.   No more restrictive provider networks

C.   Attorneys:

    1.   Tort Reform

        a.   Caps for pain and suffering

        b.   Police themselves via a "practical" new definition of frivolous suit, with reasonable penalties if all 3 criteria are met

D.   Patients (Below age 65):

    1.   Shop price and quality

    2.   Pay something for each piece of healthcare no matter

how little

3. Have a "Living Will"

4. Second opinions for non-urgent care over a "patient's selected" threshold amount

E. Hospitals:

1. Post all fees and expect to compete on price and quality.

2. Establish and run outreach clinics funded via a fund called "Uninsured Fund." See detailed plan.

F. Government:

1. Define terms (urgent, non-urgent, and catastrophic care) and regulate system as provided by this new legislation and not beyond

2. Leave Medicare ALONE!

3. Proportionally fund two pools of funds along with substantial contributions from insurance companies and state government, etc.

   a. Uninsured pool

   b. Catastrophic pool

4. Expand COBRA and health savings plans

5. Transparency for all health related revenue sources

The Carpathia Health Plan

The Rescue Healthcare Delivery System for America

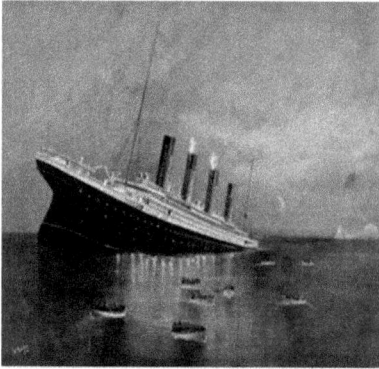
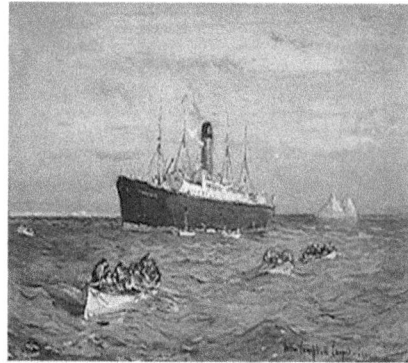

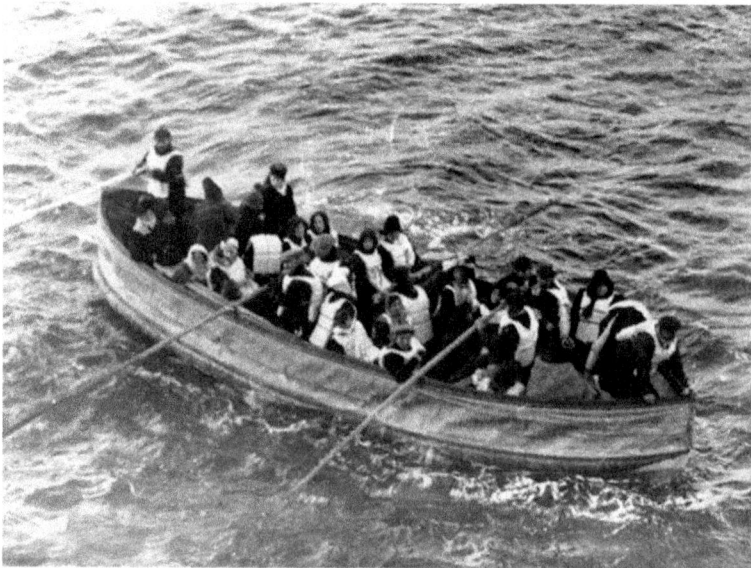

Robert Dennis, MD

The Carpathia Rescue Plan

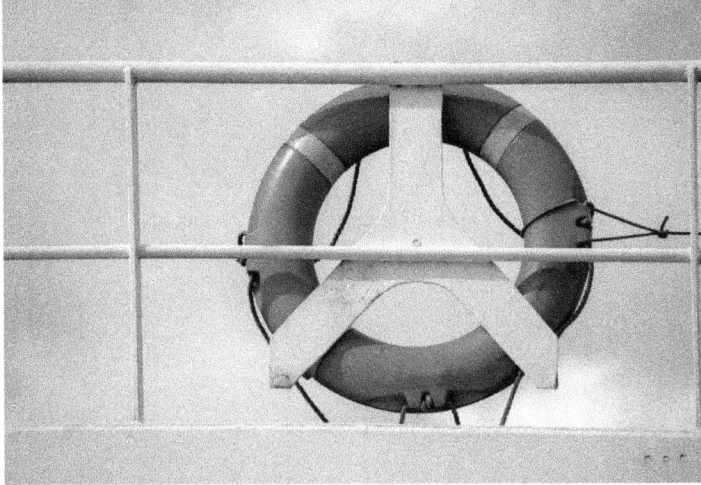

Destination = Home

Sustainable Lower Costs

A lifeboat seat for everyone: with and without pre-existing conditions, for rich and poor.

For additional information, the latest news, and other updates, please visit our website.

www.carpathiahealthplan.com